THE POLITICS OF MEDICARE

Second Edition

SOCIAL INSTITUTIONS AND SOCIAL CHANGE

An Aldine de Gruyter Series of Texts and Monographs

EDITED BY James D. Wright

V. L. Bengtson and W. A. Achenbaum, **The Changing Contract Across Generations**

Thomas G. Blomberg and Stanley Cohen (eds.), **Punishment and Social Control: Essays in Honor of Sheldon L. Messinger**

M. E. Colten and S. Gore (eds.), **Adolescent Stress: Causes and Consequences**

Rand D. Conger and Glen H. Elder, Jr., **Families in Troubled Times: Adapting to Change in Rural America**

Joel A. Devine and James D. Wright, **The Greatest of Evils: Urban Poverty and the American Underclass**

G. William Domhoff, **The Power Elite and the State: How Policy is Made in America**

G. William Domhoff, **State Autonomy or Class Dominance: Case Studies on Policy Making in America**

Paula S. England, **Comparable Worth: Theories and Evidence**

Paula S. England, **Theory on Gender/Feminism on Theory**

R. G. Evans, M. L. Barer, and T.R. Marmor, **Why Are Some People Healthy and Others Not? The Determinants of Health of Populations**

George Farkas, **Human Capital or Cultural Capitol? Ethnicity and Poverty Groups in an Urban School District**

Joseph Galaskiewicz and Wolfgang Bielefeld, **Nonprofit Organizations in an Age of Uncertainty: A Study in Organizational Change**

Davita Silfen Glasberg and Dan Skidmore, **Corporate Welfare Policy and the Welfare State: Bank Deregulation and the Savings and Loan Bailout**

Ronald F. Inglehart, Neil Nevitte, Miguel Basañez, **The North American Trajectory: Cultural, Economic, and Political Ties among the United States, Canada, and Mexico**

Gary Kleck, **Point Blank: Guns and Violence in America**

Gary Kleck, **Targeting Guns: Firearms and Their Control** (paperback)

James R. Kluegel, David S. Mason, and Bernd Wegener (eds.), **Social Justice and Political Change: Public Opinion in Capitalist and Post-Communist States**

Theodore R. Marmor, **The Politics of Medicare (Second Edition)**

Thomas S. Moore, **The Disposable Work Force: Worker Displacement and Employment Instability in America**

Clark McPhail, **The Myth of the Madding Crowd**

James T. Richardson, Joel Best, and David G. Bromley (eds.), **The Satanism Scare**

Alice S. Rossi and Peter H. Rossi, **Of Human Bonding: Parent-Child Relations Across the Life Course**

Peter H. Rossi and Richard A. Berk, **Just Punishments: Federal Guidelines and Public Views Compared**

Joseph F. Sheley and James D. Wright, **In the Line of Fire: Youth, Guns, and Violence in Urban America**

David G. Smith, **Paying for Medicare: The Politics of Reform**

Les G. Whitbeck and Dan R. Hoyt, **Nowhere to Grow: Homeless and Runaway Adolescents and Their Families**

James D. Wright, **Address Unknown: The Homeless in America**

James D. Wright and Peter H. Rossi, **Armed and Considered Dangerous: A Survey of Felons and Their Firearms, (Expanded Edition)**

James D. Wright, Peter H. Rossi, and Kathleen Daly, **Under the Gun: Weapons, Crime, and Violence in America**

Mary Zey, **Banking on Fraud: Drexel, Junk Bonds, and Buyouts**

THE POLITICS
OF MEDICARE

Second Edition

Theodore R. Marmor

ALDINE DE GRUYTER
New York

About the Author

THEODORE R. MARMOR teaches politics and public policy in Yale University's management and law schools as well as in its political science department. Educated at
Harvard and Oxford, Marmor has written widely about the politics of the modern
welfare state, and has served on a number of governmental commissions and
scholarly editorial boards. Among his numerous publications, he is the author
of *Understanding Health Care Reform* (1994) and the coauthor of *America's
Misunderstood Welfare State* (1992).

ALDINE DE GRUYTER
A division of Walter de Gruyter, Inc.
200 Saw Mill River Road
Hawthorne, New York 10532

This publication is printed on acid free paper ⊛

Library of Congress Cataloging-in-Publication Data
Marmor, Theodore R.
    The politics of Medicare/Theodore R. Marmor.—2nd ed.
      p. cm.—(Social institutions and social change)
    Includes bibliographical references and index.
    ISBN 0-202-30399-3 (cloth : alk. paper)—ISBN 0-202-30425-6 (paper : alk. paper)
      1. Medicare—Political aspects. I. Title. II. Series.

RA412.3.M37 1999
368.4′26′00973—dc21

                           99-052364

Manufactured in the United States of America
10 9 8 7 6 5 4 3 2

To the members of the "Seminar without Walls"

Contents

Preface to the Second Edition   xi

Acknowledgments   xv

Preface to the First Edition   xix

Introduction   xxiii

PART I   THE ORIGINS AND ENACTMENTS   1

1   **The Origins of the Medicare Strategy**   3
         Twentieth-Century Medicine:
             The Paradoxes of Progress   3
         Origins of the Government Health Insurance Issue   4
         Universal Health Insurance Proposals in the Fair Deal   6
         The Politics of Incrementalism:
             Turning toward the Aged   10
         The Appeal of Focusing on the Aged   11
         Focusing on Social Security Contributors   15
         Pressure Groups and Medicare:
             The Lobbying of Millions   17

2   **The Politics of Legislative Impossibility**   23
         Medicare under a Republican President   23
         The Forand Bill versus the Welfare Approach   25
         Kerr-Mills Bill of 1960   27

3   **The Politics of Legislative Possibility**   31
         Medicare, 1961   31

The Obstacle Course in Congress:
    First Try with Ways and Means   32
The Southern Democrats   35
The Kennedy Administration versus the AMA   38
Medicare's Near Miss, 1964   41

4   **The Politics of Legislative Certainty**   **45**
The Impact of the Election of 1964   45
The Administration's Proposal: H.R. 1 and S. 1   46
The Ways and Means Committee and the House
    Take Action: January–April   47
H.R. 6675 Passes the Senate: April–July   53
Medicare Comes out of the Conference Committee:
    July 26, 1965   55
The Outcome of 1965: Explanation and Issues   56

5   **Medicare and the Analysis of Social Policy in**
      American Politics   **63**
Case Studies and Cumulative Knowledge   63
Conceptual Models and the Medicare Case   64
The Origins of Medicare:
    The Rational Actor Model   64
The Responses of Medicare, 1952–64:
    The Organizational Process Model   67
The 1965 Legislation:
    The Bureaucratic Politics Model   69
Processes and Policy in American Politics:
    The Case of Medicare   71
Medicare and the Character of
    American Social Policy   80

6   **Legislation to Operation**   **87**

PART II   **THE POLITICS OF MEDICARE: 1966–99**   **93**

7   **Medicare's Politics: 1966–90**   **95**
The Origins of Medicare Revisited   95

The Politics of Accommodation:
  Medicare's Implementation and Subsequent Evolution
  from 1966 to 1970   96
The 1970s: Ineffectual Reforms and
  Intermittent Progress   99
The 1980s: The Challenge of the Reagan Era   107
Conclusion   115

8 **The Politics of Medicare Reform in the 1990s:**
   Budget Struggles, National Health Reform,
   and Shifting Conflicts   **123**
   Introduction: The Changing Context of
     Medicare's Politics in the 1990s   123
   Medicare and the 1992 Elections:
     The Reawakening of Concerns   124
   A Negative Consensus on Health Reform   126
   The 1995 Trustees' Report and Claims of Insolvency   135
   From Legislative Impasse 1995–96 to Medicare
     "Reform" in 1997   137
   The Medicare Reforms of 1997: Understanding
     the Politics of Balancing Budgets   141
   Medicare Flip-Flop   147

9 **The Ideological Context of Medicare's Politics:**
   The Presumptions of Medicare's Founders versus
   the Rise of Procompetitive Ideas in Medical Care   **151**
   Introduction   151
   Medicare's Philosophical Roots: Social Insurance
     and the Presumption of Expansion   152
   The Rise of Procompetitive Ideas about Medical Care   157

10 **Reflections on Medicare's Politics: Puzzles and Patterns** **171**
   Introduction   171
   Understanding Medicare's Politics:
     Patterns, Puzzles, and Explanatory Approaches   171
   Puzzle One: Structural Explanations
     and Medicare's Limited Evolution   173
   Puzzle Two: Insider Politics, Medicare's Price Controls,
     and the Puzzles of the Reagan/Bush Era   175

Puzzle Three: Medicare 1995–99—Macro Politics
    and the Emergence of Unexpected Remedies   176
Conclusion   179

Medicare Scholarship: A Selective Review Essay   183

Glossary   193

References to Part I   207

References to Part II   213

Index   221

Preface to the Second Edition

U nderstanding Medicare's origins was the central subject of the first edition of this book. Part I is a straightforward reprinting of the 1973 edition except for some minor adjustments in the order of what was initially the epilogue and the conclusion. I decided to leave the original study as it was for two reasons. First, there has been relatively little new scholarship on Medicare's enactment since the flurry of books in the late 1960s and early 1970s. What scholarship has emerged is discussed in this edition's expanded bibliographical essay. But the limited volume of this commentary on Medicare does not fully explain why I was so disinclined to rewrite the early chapters. The fundamental rationale is really quite simple. The scholarship published on Medicare's enactment politics has not challenged any major interpretation of the book and, accordingly, it seemed needless to change what was a settled narrative.

Part I's Medicare story answers one set of questions. How could the American political system yield a policy that simultaneously appeased widely held antigovernment biases and yet used the federal government to provide major social insurance entitlement? How was one particularly strong interest group—the AMA—overcome legislatively and yet placated enough to participate in Medicare? Most of all, how did the Medicare law emerge so enlarged from the earlier proposals that themselves had occasioned such controversy?

The second edition's Part II tells a different kind of story. It deals with what happened to Medicare politically as it turned from a legislative act in 1965–66 to a major program of American government in the three decades since. Part II both characterizes the trends and shocks that have marked Medicare's operational politics, and reflects on what explains them. Its subject, then, is the politics of Medicare since enactment, emphasizing the form, salience, and significance of those politics over time.

Medicare's anniversaries illustrate the changing place of the program in American politics since 1966. Little attention was paid to Medicare on its tenth anniversary in 1976 as other issues crowded the public agenda. A decade later, Medicare was celebrated as a Republican president (and most American political leaders) steered clear of the more controversial issue of national health insurance. By 1996—the thirtieth anniversary—Medicare was front-page news, the object of a partisan presidential battle reminiscent of Medicare's place in the presidential election of 1964.

The story of Part II thus raises a new set of questions about Medicare for a different set of actors, both new and old. What has been its role in the extraordinarily complicated political and economic world of American medicine? What was Medicare's connection to the disputes over persistent medical inflation in the decades after 1966 and the efforts to contain medical costs? (In 1998 the 14 percent of gross national product expended on medical care represented a more than twofold increase in three decades.) How did Medicare's political salience vary with the cycles of attention and inattention to the controversial topic of national health insurance? More broadly, throughout the whole period of 1996–99, to what extent was Medicare's political fate shaped by broader forces in the environment as opposed to the developments within its narrower medical care domain?

Unlike Part I, Part II interprets the historical record rather than describing in detail the episodes constituting that history. Of the existing scholarly commentary on the Medicare program in operation, very little addresses its politics and few of the published political analyses review the program's implementation comprehensively. Chapters 7 and 8 aim to provide narrative accounts of Medicare's controversies over the period 1966–99, while also portraying the program's changing place in American politics. Chapter 9 is quite different in aim and structure. It characterizes the shifting ideological context in which Medicare's politics were situated in the decades following enactment, first discussing the fate of the aspirations for expanding Medicare into national health insurance and then describing the growth of procompetitive ideas in American politics. The final chapter 10 reflects on some of the major puzzles about Medicare's past and discusses a variety of conceptual frameworks for resolving them. It is a counterpart to chapter 5's commentary on Medicare's enactment, more analytical than narrative in character. The new edition closes with an extensive bibliographical essay on Medicare and a glossary of specialized terms.

It is important to be candid about what this book does not do. It does not, for example, explain either the timing or the technical character of program innovations like Diagnosis-Related Groups (DRGs), the prospective hospital payment method introduced in 1983. Nor does it explore how elderly and disabled Americans actually experience Medicare's administration. This is a topic few scholars have addressed, but which advocates for the elderly understand quite well. Moreover, it does not review the topics that dominate the pages of health services journals—questions such as the effects of one or another policy innovation on access, costs, or quality. This edition also does not address two of the topics that have been central to Medicare's internal reform aspirations in the 1990s: the program's emphasis on combatting fraud both in rhetoric and practice, and the managerial restructuring Bruce Vladeck launched when heading the Health Care Financing Agency. Both are worthy topics of undoubted political importance, the antifraud campaign because it became such a key feature of public attention, and the reorganization because it illustrated the micropolitics of how an agency responds to efforts to reduce its role.

The process of producing the new book was both extended in time and indirect. I considered revising the original edition at many points since 1973. Though the first edition remained in print, its subject obviously grew more distant and some teachers who continued to use it in classes urged me to update the study. Reflecting over time on Medicare's policy disputes and political struggles, I continued to publish on various topics. Chapters 7 through 10 incorporate substantial portions of these articles, which is acknowledged in the endnotes.

One other development crucially aided the completion of this second edition. I had agreed to be a visiting professor at the Kennedy School of Government in the fall of 1996, but had not worked out what I would teach. A chance conversation with Graham Allison, an old friend from graduate student days, revealed that he too was revising a book published in the 1970s. We agreed to give a seminar on both the Cuban missile crisis and the politics of Medicare, using that format to present what we wanted to include in the revised second editions of our book. Allison, with his coauthor Philip Zelikow, finished his revision in 1998, a competitive move for which I have only recently forgiven him. I want to thank Graham warmly, reflecting with pleasure on that collegial experiment, one that is as rare as is the revisions of books published twenty-five years earlier.

Acknowledgments

In completing this new edition, I have incurred a number of debts that are a pleasure to acknowledge. I thought about a second edition repeatedly, especially in the late 1980s. At that time Professor Norman Daniels urged me to reflect on Medicare for a special issue of a philosophy and medicine journal and that prompted me to summarize my views in ways that would later prove helpful in this revision. I am very grateful to Daniels for the stimulus to reflect and the publishing outlet.

In completing the early drafts of what are now chapters 7 through 10, I have relied on the help of a number of helpful, competent assistants, many of them postdoctoral fellows at Yale. Carlos Cano spent 1991–92 making the transition from psychiatrist to policy analyst and, as a postdoctoral fellow, worked hard to make what is now chapter 8 empirically reliable and stylistically compatible with the first edition. A government official at the Department of Health and Human Services through the 1990s, Cano has my warm thanks for the tireless efforts he made to improve this work. Another former graduate student, Jon Oberlander, made his dissertation subject the topics I have tried to address in Part II. He has become over time a valued coauthor, a constant source of stimulation and oversight, and the single most important influence on my thinking about what Medicare's politics became since 1966. I am enormously in his debt. The same is true for those closer to day-to-day writing. Victoria Bilski, in addition to administering the postdoctoral program for which I am responsible, has regularly improved my prose with her editing skills. Elizabeth Esty, a lawyer turned policy analyst, joined the team in October of 1998, rather late in the process. But she is the one whose determination to help me finish this book by something close to the publisher's deadline actually made it happen. Without her knowledge of medical care, her analytical and editing skills, and her willingness to be an "enforcer," this book would not have appeared in this millennium. I gratefully acknowledge her decisive assistance. Camille Costelli, my office assistant, created in 1998–99 an environment in which this writing—and much other work—could be accomplished with more civility and reliability than could be accurately described as the norm. She deserves and has my gratitude.

My most profound debts, however, are to the circle of colleagues who have been my intellectual companions over the past decades in the field of health politics, policy, and law. Mostly but not exclusively former students, they constitute the audience likely to care most about what I write and, in that sense, have been the most powerful stimulant to finishing work like this second edition. I have already mentioned Jon Oberlander, who is himself a member of this seminar without walls. Professor James Morone of Brown University, long ago a graduate student of mine at the University of Chicago, has for a quarter century been a leader in this seminar. He has both written works that advanced the understanding of Medicare and prompted me to continue my own scholarship on the topic. Professor Joseph White, not a former student and a relative newcomer to the field, has contributed greatly to my education about the politics of budgets and the mix of sense and nonsense in contemporary fiscal debates. I am delighted to acknowledge his help, as I am in connection with the reading of this manuscript by Mark Peterson, Professor of Politics and Public Policy at UCLA and editor of *The Journal of Health Politics, Policy & Law*. He, like White, went over drafts of what became chapters 8 and 9 with a degree of care, candor, and concise criticism that was remarkable and much appreciated. Jerry Mashaw, my Yale colleague and coauthor on so many works, limited his contributions on *The Politics of Medicare* to reading early drafts of the new chapters. But, if the scope of his review was bordered, the clarity and force of his critical observations were considerable. The revisions would have stopped sooner had it not been for the stimulus of his reactions. In this, as in many other ways, he remains my closest intellectual companion, someone I have been very lucky to have had so near for two decades.

Two others in the "seminar without walls" have been terribly helpful in recent years and deserve thanks, even though their assistance has been concentrated less on *Medicare* revisions than on other tasks that might have deflected me from finishing this edition. Jacob Hacker has turned from graduate student to coauthor and colleague with an ease that is remarkable and with benefits to me that have been quite considerable. While finishing this revision, he took the lead in completing another assignment we had taken on—a dissection of the fads and fashions of managerial commentary in contemporary American medical politics that both influenced chapter 10 and, because of his efforts, did not require from me as much time as expected. I thank him for that help and for the delight his own intellectual development has brought to me, his former teacher. Lastly, there is Larry Jacobs, whose work on public opinion has stimulated my thinking greatly, as the bibliographical essay demonstrates. But his greatest contribution for this book was to take the lead in completing our common project on the political paradoxes that the Oregon Health plan—and its reception—illustrate. Here, too, the "seminar" participants were at work, with Jacobs and Oberlander as my coauthors in a scholarly essay that was finished in 1998 and freed me up to complete this book. Anyone who has lived a busy scholarly life knows that one's work is never as individualistic as title pages suggest. It is not false modesty to say that my scholarly career would have been very much less "productive" without the intellectual exchange and the emotional support of these seminarians.

There are others whose assistance has been very valuable and much appreciated. My Yale colleague Mark Goldberg was willing to read the last drafts of chapters in Part II and saved them from a number of errors. For that, and other comradely efforts, I am very grateful to Mark. Eliot Fishman and John Pakutka helped in final reviews of the book's documentation and in preparing the charts that appear in Part II. I am thankful for their assistance and especially grateful to Paul Conrad, the *Los Angeles Times* regular cartoonist, for giving me permission to use his work in my work.

For financial help at a crucial time I am much indebted to Jim Knickman of the Robert Wood Johnson Foundation. He found a flexible and timely form of a grant to "plan" and to begin the process of revising this book. That was in the early 1990s and, though the time this process took stretched beyond his and my imagination, the grant was in fact crucial. Lastly, there is Richard Koffler to thank, the editor of Aldine de Gruyter, whose participation has been essential to the production of this second edition. Richard has displayed a degree of patience in waiting for this manuscript that calls Job to mind. To say that he has retained faith in the project's completion is to engage in considerable understatement. On April 24, 1992, Koffler warned me that "if nothing can be done [to complete the book], we gnash our teeth and postpone publication until '93." That was, no doubt, one of the least prescient publishing comments he has ever made. However, I am the fortunate one and want to thank Richard for bearing with this project while Medicare—and my life—took turns in the 1990s we could only dimly imagine in 1992. I am both gratified and grateful that he appears genuinely pleased with the result of what could be called "the long wait."

My wife Jan, the real coauthor of the first edition, relieved herself of
any obligation for this publication but relished its completion. She
deserves credit for whatever grace the first edition's writing exhibited.
I want to dedicate this edition, however, to the members of the "seminar without walls."

Preface to the First Edition

I want to explain the nature of this book and, especially, to alert the readers as to what they may expect in the concluding part, chapter 6.* The first five chapters constitute a case study of Medicare politics. This study is not intended to provide a full history of the origins, evolution, enactment, and consequences of Medicare. Those interested in a fuller account of this long, complicated episode in policymaking should consult the studies by Harris, Somers and Somers, and Feingold listed in the bibliographical citations. But neither is this book merely an isolated case study of one important social policy in the United States. Rather, it is both a detailed case study and an attempt to contribute more broadly to cumulative knowledge of U.S. politics and public policy. While these broader concerns are expressed throughout, they are most explicitly raised in the final chapter.

Case studies inevitably mix the peculiar and the typical, the general and the specific, the thematic and the descriptive. By focusing on one decision, one set of government actions, one policy issue, the case analyst cannot "prove" generalizations, but he can comment upon generalizations about politics in at least three useful ways.

First, case studies may be evaluated as instances of particular analytic methods. The notion that such methods lead to selective (and, by implication, biased) analysis can be explicitly evaluated in particular monographs. By reviewing the implicit framework of the study, one can show the respects in which the questions posed, the answers given, and the implications drawn would have differed in other analytic schemes. Such conceptual discussion is important for cumulative work in any discipline; it is the precondition to sustained generalizations from individual studies. Only when units of analysis are the same, central con-

---

*Now Chapter 5 for the present edition. *Ed.*

cepts analogous, and inference patterns similar can social scientists "sum up" the descriptions, explanations, and predictions of a number of case studies. Hence, the first respect in which a case study has general relevance (for cumulative effort) is in the explicit discussion of its conceptual framework and the difference such a framework makes in the particular study.

Second, case studies can illustrate some of the problems and prospects of procedural generalizations about political behavior. We have no lack of assertions about how the American political system operates, how public opinion is formed, how concerns become political issues, how legislatures and legislators, executive agencies and executive officials operate in their environments. What we need in many instances is the detailed explication of the connection between such summary generalizations and the innumerable studies of individual instances of political action. A monograph on Medicare—one of the most important post–World War II social policy issues—can be used to illustrate explicitly what seem to be promising generalizations.

Third, case studies can offer important instances of who gets what in the U.S. political system. They can, in short, be used to illustrate generalizations about the substantive content (the benefits and burdens) of U.S. domestic policy. It should perhaps be stressed that Medicare's distribution of benefits and burdens *need* not be typical of domestic, social welfare, or even health policies in the United States. But one can review the Medicare outcome from this substantive-policy standpoint and thus begin to extend the significance of this particular occurrence in American public policy.

All of this can be done without falsely claiming a case study is more than a detailed analysis of how a government behaves in a particular instance. Cumulation of knowledge about U.S. politics will not proceed unless analysts explicitly discuss the conceptual, procedural, and substantive implications of the cases they study.

This book, though not a full history, ranges over the history of Medicare disputes. Three central questions guide its organization and selection of detail. First, why did Medicare arise as a political issue at the time and in the form it did (chap. 1)? The problem is to account for the timing and character of the public policy initiatives we have come to term *Medicare*. The second problem is to describe and account for the pattern of responses to Medicare initiatives over time. The three types of responses include: the nature of the public debate over governmental health insurance for the aged; the kind of group conflict that characterized Medicare; and the sequence of bureaucratic proposals and congressional reactions in the 1952–64 period (chap. 2 and 3). Thirdly, I am

interested in explaining the outcome of this intense social policy struggle. The output of the Congress—the Medicare statute of 1965—is the
subject of chapter 4. In addition, I set out some of the lessons and issues
surrounding the enactment of Medicare, and conclude the narrative by
discussing some of the operational problems which arose the first year,
and subsequent issues—most prominently the cost increases—bring
the book up to the present debate over national health insurance. The
chapter on "Medicare and the Analysis of Social Policy" departs from the
sequential organization and reviews the conceptual, procedural, and
substantive significance of the Medicare case. Those primarily interested in the policymaking process might benefit by beginning with this
chapter and then referring back to the preceding text.

This American edition carries over the form of documentation used
in the English edition (Routledge and Kegan Paul, London, 1970). Citations in the text, indicated by author's name and year of publication,
are fully documented in the Bibliographical citations section. Following
the Citations there is a more general discussion of sources for the study
and suggestions for further reading. The Glossary provides further
explanation of unfamiliar terms used to describe the legislative process
and the medical care and health insurance industries and a list of institutional names used.

Three institutions have provided support for initial research and
forums for criticism of earlier drafts: The Harvard University program
in the Economics and Administration of Medical Care; Harvard's John
Fitzgerald Kennedy School of Government; and the University of Wisconsin's Institute for Research on Poverty. I want to express my gratitude for such support without in any way holding these institutions
responsible for my conclusions.

Full acknowledgment to those who provided valuable and appreciated assistance can be found in the discussion of sources. Jan Marmor
was as much coauthor of this book as chief research assistant. Her editing has guided the final form of the text and, in many places, her writing has supplied the final version. I want to thank especially the former
Secretary of Health, Education, and Welfare, Wilbur Cohen. This study
could not have been written without the extraordinary access to primary materials I enjoyed as his special assistant in the summer of 1966.
Few young scholars are permitted to investigate the files of political
leaders still in the midst of public life. Even fewer are given the freedom
I was given to publish the conclusions they draw from such encounters.
No one who reads this book will find a slavish devotion to any of my
sources, but I feel particularly appreciative to former Secretary Cohen
for extending to me the kind of educational opportunity his own

teacher—Edwin Witte, the late secretary to President Roosevelt's Committee on Economic Security—extended to him in the heyday of the New Deal.

Allan Sindler, the editor of a volume on *American Political Institutions and Public Policy* in which a shorter version of this study first appeared, helped more than he realized in making this study more readable. Carol Mermey and Nordis Nesset deserve special mention for so efficiently helping put together the final version of this book for both its English and U.S. editions.

Introduction

On July 30, 1965, President Johnson flew to Independence, Missouri, to sign the Medicare bill in the presence of former president Harry S. Truman. The new statute—technically Title 18 of the Social Security Amendments of 1965—included two related insurance programs to finance substantial portions of the hospital and physician expenses incurred by Americans over the age of 65. The bill-signing ceremony in Missouri was attended by scores of government officials, health leaders, and private citizens, many of whom had participated in the long, bitter fight for social security health insurance during the administrations of presidents Roosevelt, Truman, Eisenhower, Kennedy, and Johnson. That afternoon, Johnson reviewed the two decades that had culminated in the Medicare legislation, and observed that the surprising thing was not "the passage of this bill . . . but that it took so many years to pass it."

President Johnson's remark underscored the obvious fact that good health, like peace and prosperity, is a laudable goal, widely shared by Americans. Yet the president was too astute a practitioner of politics to be really surprised by the delay in devising an acceptable federal health insurance program. Public attempts to improve American health standards have typically precipitated bitter debate, even as the issue has shifted from the professional and legal status of physicians to the availability of hospital care, from quackery among doctors and druggists to the provision of public health programs. The beginning of the American Medical Association itself (1847) was part of the broader effort to define the legitimate medical practitioner and to raise the educational standards expected of him. Later in the nineteenth century, licensing of physicians by the states and the regulation of drugs became political issues as the AMA conducted campaigns against medical charlatans and pharmaceutical quackery. Hospital care, once almost exclusively supported by private institutions, became politically controversial once general hospitals grew with the support of local tax funds. Sanitation measures, disease control through mass inoculation, state regulation of hospitals—all commanded increasing public attention as Americans left the countryside to congregate in large urban centers after the Civil War.

It was not until the twentieth century, however, that medical care problems, always of concern to local government, generated interest in national politics. That interest, particularly in the period after World War II, focused on three features of the American system of medical care: medical research, hospital construction, and federal health insurance programs. Since 1945, the federal government massively increased its support of medical research (primarily through the National Institutes of Health, the research arm of the Public Health Service), and under the Hill- Burton Act of 1946, subsidized a significant portion (25–30 percent) of the nation's postwar hospital construction (Somers and Somers, 1961, 50). By 1964, federal, state, and local governments together expended almost $7 billion of the $35.4 billion Americans spent in that year for health services. "In few fields," concluded the *Congressional Quarterly,* "were there more new federal programs established in the postwar era, or more significant changes made, than in health" (1965a, 1113).

Americans were no less concerned about expanding the federal government's role in providing health insurance, but in this controversial area postwar government action did not parallel the rapid expansion of support for research and hospital facilities. The inaction persisted despite public sentiment to the contrary. Opinion surveys from 1943 to 1965 indicated a relatively stable two-thirds majority of Americans favoring some government assistance in the financing of personal health services (Peters, 1964, 38; Cantril, 1952, 439–44; Hamilton, 1972). As proposals became more specific, the public usually showed a less favorable response to any particular method. Yet by 1965, the Gallup pollsters reported, "Sixty-three percent approve of the compulsory medical insurance program soon to be considered by the 89th Congress" (Gallup, 1965).

The legislative activity of the U.S. Congress, however, is never simply a matter of ratifying public opinion polls. For controversial legislation to be enacted, proponents must be sufficiently organized to make their views felt. There must be some agreement on "remedies" to bolster the public acknowledgment of health "problems." Beyond that, the support of executive agencies is normally required in framing and presenting complex legislative proposals. Bills must have sponsors and floor-managers in both houses of the Congress, and they must pass through a maze of obstacles: committee hearings, placement on the agenda by the House Rules Committee, votes in both houses, and if successfully passed, a conference committee in which differences between House and Senate versions are ironed out. It was not until 1965 that a health insurance bill for the aged emerged from the congressional process to become public law. Understanding how that bill became law illustrates some of the typical patterns by which divisive public issues run the course in American politics from initial demand to statutory enactment.

I

THE ORIGINS AND ENACTMENTS

1

The Origins of the Medicare Strategy

TWENTIETH-CENTURY MEDICINE: THE PARADOXES OF PROGRESS

In 1912, a distinguished Harvard professor called attention to the remarkable advances in medical science, technology, and therapy that Americans could look forward to enjoying. That year, Professor Lawrence Henderson remarked, constituted a "Great Divide" when "for the first time in human history, a random patient with a random disease consulting a doctor chosen at random stands a better than 50/50 chance of benefitting from the encounter" (Harris, 1966, 5). Twentieth-century developments have fully borne out this prediction that the health industry would have much to offer the consumers of its services. One by one, dread diseases—T.B., cholera, diphtheria, pneumonia, smallpox, polio—have been controlled. Surgical and drug therapy have dramatically reduced the impact of diseases and maladies that preventive medicine has not conquered. These changes, along with substantial improvements in the general American standard of living, have not resulted in diminished illness, but they have startlingly altered mortality rates. The newborn child in 1900 had a life expectancy of 47 years; by 1965 the average was 70 years. These improvements are, however, just one side of what Herman and Anne Somers have called "the paradox of medical progress" (1961, 4, 7). Not only has medical progress increased the proportion of old people in the population, but "as we preserve life at all age levels there is more enduring disability for the population as a whole" (ibid.).

The demand for medical care has increased both through improved capacity and heightened expectations among longer-living populations. Changes in the organization of medical care have accompanied the rapid increase in utilization. Since 1930, the average number of patient visits to the doctor has more than doubled, increasing from 2.6 to 5.3

visits per year. The type of doctors Americans visit has changed in the process. Whereas in 1930 two-thirds of American physicians were general practitioners, three decades later two-thirds were specialists (HEW, 1959, 26–29). The site of the most complicated medical activity has shifted to the hospital.

With these shifts the costs of medical activities have steadily increased. Between 1953 and 1963, expenditures for all health services more than doubled. The price of hospital beds rose 90 percent, while physicians' fees increased 37 percent. The mean expenditure of American families for medical care during this decade grew by 70 percent. Figures on mean expenditures fail to show, however, the uneven distribution of illness throughout the society, and its financial implications. "Much of the total use of health services," a 1967 study concluded, "is accounted for by the relatively small proportion of the population with serious illness episodes"; people with illness "requiring hospitalization account for one-half of all private expenditures, but amount to only 8 percent of the population" (Anderson and Anderson, 1967, 122ff.).

The combination of increased medical competence, heightened consumer expectations and utilization, and rising costs has shaped the environment for public policy demands. But these experiences, common to Western industrial countries, have not predetermined either the proposals for government action or their fate. Bismarck's Germany initiated health insurance for industrial workers as early as 1883; England in 1911 incorporated health insurance for low-income workers into a social security program providing pensions, unemployment compensation, and sickness benefits. By 1940, no Western European country was without a government health insurance program for at least its low-income workers, though there were substantial differences in beneficiaries, benefits, governmental financing, and regulatory mechanisms. The enactment of Medicare in 1965 illustrated America's comparatively late entry into compulsory health insurance, and its restriction to the aged alone was quite unlike the patterns established in other Western industrial countries.

ORIGINS OF THE GOVERNMENT
HEALTH INSURANCE ISSUE

Demands in America for government involvement in health insurance date back to the first decade of the twentieth century. The impetus in these early efforts came from academics, lawyers, and other professionals, organized in the American Association for Labor Legislation (AALL). During the years 1915–18, this group made a concerted effort to shepherd its model medical care insurance bill through several state legislatures, but with no success. The American Medical Association (AMA), whose officials had initially cooperated with the AALL, found local medical societies adamantly opposed to the state health insurance bills, and in 1920 the AMA House of Delegates announced

> its opposition to the institution of any plan embodying the system of compulsory contributory insurance against illness, or any other plan of compulsory insurance which provides for medical service to be rendered contributors or their dependents, provided, controlled, or regulated by any state or Federal government. (Feingold, 1966, 89)

Even more disappointing to the labor health insurance reformers was the unequivocal opposition to the model bills of Samuel Gompers, the president of the American Federation of Labor, who feared that any form of compulsory social insurance would serve as an excuse for government control of working men. The strength of the opposition prevented America from following England's example of insuring low-income workers against illness. During the 1920s, a variety of groups undertook studies of health care financing in the United States, and attention turned to the feasibility of group medical practice and of prepayment medical plans. But it was not until the Great Depression in an atmosphere of general concern for economic insecurity that a sustained interest in government health insurance reappeared. The evolution of the 1965 Medicare Act reaches back to this New Deal period. To understand the particular form of the Medicare legislation, and to explain the two decades of controversy and delay at which President Johnson expressed surprise, one must begin the analysis here.

The source of renewed interest in government health insurance was President Roosevelt's advisory Committee on Economic Security, created in 1934 to draft a social security bill providing a minimum income for the aged, the unemployed, the blind, and the widowed and their children. The result was the Social Security bill of 1935, which, in addition to providing for insurance against loss of income, broached the subject of a government health insurance program. Edwin Witte, a former professor of economics at the University of Wisconsin who was executive director of the committee, described the extent of the committee's involvement with health insurance and the critical response of the AMA:

> When in 1934 the Committee on Economic Security announced that it was studying health insurance, it was at once subjected to misrepresentation and vilification. In the original social security bill there was one line to the effect that the Social Security Board should study the problem

and make a report to Congress. That little line was responsible for so
many telegrams to the members of Congress that the entire social security program seemed endangered until the Ways and Means Committee
unanimously struck it out of the bill. (Feingold, 1966, 91)

Roosevelt's fears that the controversial issue of government health
insurance would jeopardize the Social Security bill and, later, his
chances for reelection, kept him from vigorously sponsoring the proposal. For many of his advisers in the Committee on Economic Security,
however, the discussions in Washington in the mid-thirties marked the
beginning of an active interest in the subject. The divorce of compulsory
health insurance from the original Social Security program of 1935
had alerted the critics within the medical world to the possibility of
attempts to enlarge the partial government program, to "get a foot-in-
the-door for socialized medicine." In response they reversed their former opposition to private health insurance alternatives: in an effort to
forestall federal action, the AMA began to endorse Blue Cross and commercial hospital insurance and, in the case of state Blue Shield plans,
actively to support private insurance plans for surgical and medical
expenses (Davis, 1941, 167–68; Burrow, 1963, 244–47, 288–89).[1] In the
meantime, passage of the Social Security Act had freed advocates of
compulsory health insurance from pressing concerns about providing
income protection for the aged, the blind, and dependent women and
children. Their attention was now directed to the broad social question
of how equitably medical care was distributed in postdepression America. From 1939 onward, their activities were reflected in the annual
introduction of congressional bills proposing compulsory health insurance for the entire population. An orphan of the New Deal, government
medical care insurance was to become one of the most prominent aspirations of Harry Truman's "Fair Deal."

UNIVERSAL HEALTH INSURANCE PROPOSALS
IN THE FAIR DEAL

Although the government health insurance issue was originally
raised in conjunction with social security income protection, New
Deal–Fair Deal champions of medical care proposals did not view it
primarily as a measure to further income security but as a remedy for
the inequitable distribution of medical services. The proponents of Truman's compulsory insurance program took for granted that financial
means should not determine the quality and quantity of medical services a citizen received. "Access to the means of attainment and preservation of health," the 1952 report of Truman's Commission on the

Health Needs of the Nation flatly stated, "is a basic human right." The health insurance problem in this view was the degree to which the use of health services varied with income (and not simply illness). In contrast, for those who considered minimum accessibility of health services a standard of adequacy, the provision of charity medicine in doctors' offices and general hospitals represented a solution, and the problem was to fill in where present charity care was unavailable.

The Truman solution to the problem of unequal accessibility to health services was to remove the financial barriers to care through government action. A radical redistribution of income was, in theory, an alternative solution, but not one that the Truman administration felt moved to advocate. Rather, as he made clear in his State of the Union message in 1948, Truman's goal was "to enact a comprehensive insurance system which would remove the money barrier between illness and therapy, . . . [and thus] protect all our people equally . . . against ill health." Bills embracing such goals had been introduced as early as 1935, but the first to receive widespread public attention was S. 1620, introduced by Senator Robert Wagner (D., N.Y.) in 1939. A decade later, during Truman's term of office, it was S. 1679 that Senator Wagner, Senator Murray (D., Mont.), and Representative Dingell (D., Mich.) presented for congressional consideration. By 1949, the introduction of a Murray-Wagner-Dingell bill had become an annual event, which was invariably followed by congressional refusal to hold hearings on the bill.

Through the decade, public opinion polls continued to report favorable reactions to federal involvement in health insurance. However, although from 1939 to 1946 the Democrats controlled both houses of Congress, the partisan Democratic majority did not make up a programmatic voting majority. On the issue of federal health insurance, there were simply too few legislative supporters to bring repeatedly introduced bills through the stages of committee hearings, committee approval, and congressional passage. By 1945, officials within the Social Security Board[2] had secured presidential endorsement of the Murray-Wagner-Dingell proposal, but the advantage of Truman's support was offset by the congressional elections the following year, which returned Republican majorities in both the House and the Senate. This Congress, it has been observed, "was generally at loggerheads with Truman in domestic affairs," and in the campaign of 1948, the president used its inaction, on health insurance and other domestic issues, to berate the "do-nothing Republican 80th Congress." The election of 1948, returning the presidency to Truman and control of the Congress to the Democrats, left Truman and his advisers with high hopes for enactment of the domestic proposals that had highlighted his Fair Deal campaign against Dewey (*Congressional Quarterly,* 1965b, 4, 7).

Early in 1949, in keeping with his recent campaign pledges, the president requested congressional action on medical care insurance. The specifications of the proposal repeated those of previous Murray-Wagner-Dingell bills:

—the insurance benefits would cover all medical, dental, hospital and nursing care expenses.

—beneficiaries would include all contributors to the plan and their dependents, and for the medical needs of a destitute minority which would not be reached by the contributory plan, provisions were made for Federal grants to the states.

—the financing mechanism would be compulsory 3 percent payroll tax divided equally between employee and employer.

—administration would be in the hands of a national health insurance board within the Federal Security Agency.

—to minimize the degree of federal control over doctors and patients, it was specified that doctors and hospitals would be free not to join the plan; patients would be free to choose their own doctors and doctors would reserve the right to reject patients whom they did not want; doctors who agreed to treat patients under the plan would be paid for their services by the national health board, and the question of whether they would be paid on a stated-fee, per capita or salary basis would be left to the majority decision of the participating practitioners in each health service area. (Kelley, 1966, 70, 71)

The bill's reception in the 81st Congress was disappointing to the Truman administration. Although the Democrats had gained 75 seats in the House, a coalition of anti-Truman Southern Democrats and Republicans blocked most of Truman's major domestic proposals. Despite some success in housing and social security legislation, the federal aid to education bill floundered, and the administration's health insurance plan was not reported out of committee in either house.

In retrospect, the 1949 campaign for universal government health insurance represented the only time such a proposal had the remotest chance of gaining congressional enactment. The Democrats had their House majority reduced from 263–171 to 235–199 in the elections of 1950, and barely maintained control of the Senate by a margin of two. Attempts to leave doctors' participation in the national health insurance plan voluntary had failed to placate the American Medical Association. The organization had been roused to a nationwide propaganda campaign, directed by the California public relations firm Whitaker and Baxter and financed by an emergency "war chest," which was raised by "taxing" every AMA member $25 (Kelley, 1966; Mayer, 1949). The doctors had enlisted hundreds of voluntary organizations and pressure groups to oppose compulsory health insurance, and their crusade was conducted on a note of hysteria, holding out horrific visions of a socialized America ruled by an autocratic federal government. Doctors displayed AMA-provided posters, which presented a color reproduction of the famous Fildes painting of the doctor at the bedside of a sick child. "Keep Politics out of this Picture!" was the accompanying caption (Kelley, 1966, 77). Ignoring the stipulations that doctors would remain free to choose their own patients, and patients to choose their own doctors, the AMA campaign pictured an impersonal medical world under the national health plan in which patients and doctors were forced unwillingly upon each other. In 1950, the AMA took the issues of "socialized medicine" to both the primary and general elections, and their propaganda was credited with the defeat of some of the Senate's firmest supporters of health insurance.

The absence of a programmatic majority in the Congress repeatedly frustrated Truman's health insurance demands. He responded with vitriolic criticism of the American Medical Association as the public's worst enemy in the effort to redistribute medical care more equitably. But the fact was that Truman could not command majorities for any of his major domestic proposals—lambasting the AMA was one way of coping with this executive-legislative stalemate.

Although Truman persisted in requesting compulsory health insurance in 1950, 1951, and 1952, his advisers agreed that after 1949 the prospects for such a broad program were bleak. Among those advisers were Federal Security Agency officials Wilbur J. Cohen and I. S. Falk,[3] two of the men who had had most to do with the drafting of health insurance proposals since 1935. Recognizing the need to "resurrect health insurance" in a dramatically new and narrower form, Cohen and Falk worked out a plan that would limit health insurance to the beneficiaries of the Old Age and Survivors Insurance program (the national, contributory, earnings-related pension program for the retired aged and their survivors, established by the Social Security Act of 1935). Oscar Ewing, head of the Federal Security Agency, considered this approach "terrific," and it shaped the entire strategy of health insurance advocates in the period after 1951. The persistent failure of Truman's health proposals had made the need for a new strategy evident; presumptions about the American public's acceptance of social security programs made the content of the new strategy appear politically feasible. Thus the stage was set in early 1951 for what has come to be called "Medicare" proposals. Millions of dollars spent on propaganda, the activation of a broad cleavage in American politics, the framing of choice in health insurance between socialism and "the voluntary way," the bitter, personally vindictive battle between Truman's supporters and the AMA-led opposition—these comprised the legacy of the fight over general health insurance and provided the setting for the emergence of Medicare as an issue.

THE POLITICS OF INCREMENTALISM:
TURNING TOWARD THE AGED

Major shifts in the demands brought to the Congress seldom derive from dispassionate analysis of contemporary social conditions. The decision to pare down President Truman's health insurance aims to a more modest hospitalization insurance program for the aged was no exception to this pattern. In 1951 and 1952, extended discussions took place among Truman's social security advisers about how to deal with congressional reluctance to enact his administration's health program. In October 1951 presidential assistant David Stowe outlined for Truman three ways of responding to the bleak legislative prospects for general health insurance: "softpedal the general health issue; push some peripheral programs in the area but not general insurance; or appoint a study commission in the area but not general insurance; or appoint a study commission to go over the whole problem." Three days later Truman accepted his staff's recommendation to create a study commission and charged them with finding "the right people" (Cornwell, 1965, 70–71). But the effort to "push some peripheral programs" had already begun, with the president's acquiescence. In June 1951, Oscar Ewing, acting on the suggestions of Cohen and Falk, announced a new plan to insure the 7 million aged social security beneficiaries for 60 days of hospital care a year. "It is difficult for me to see," said Ewing to an assembled corps of reporters, "how anyone with a heart can oppose this [type of program]" (Harris, 1966, 55).

Ewing, Cohen, and Falk assumed the administration could most easily build an issue majority in the Congress by narrowing previous demands and tailoring them to meet the objections of critical congressmen and pressure groups. The major objections to the Truman health program that the Medicare strategists felt they had to meet included charges that: (1) general medical insurance was a "give-away" program, which made no distinction between the deserving and undeserving poor; (2) it would substantially help too many well-off Americans who did not need financial assistance; (3) it would swell utilization of existing medical services beyond their capacity; and (4) it would produce excessive federal control of physicians, constituting a precedent for socialism in America. In connection with the latter objection, there was the widespread fear, grounded in the bitter, hostile propaganda of the AMA, that physicians would refuse to provide services under a national health insurance program.

To meet these objections, the proponents of "peripheral programs" turned from the health problems of the general population to those of the aged. As a group, the aged could be presumed to be both needy and deserving because, through no fault of their own, they had lower earning capacity and higher medical expenses than any other adult age group. Since the proponents wished to avoid imposition of a means test to determine eligibility within the ranks of the aged, they limited the beneficiaries to those persons over 65 (and their spouses) who had contributed to the social security system during their working life. As an additional advance concession to spike the guns of those opponents who could be counted on to assault the program as a "give-away," benefits were limited to 60 days of hospital care. Finally, physician services were excluded from the plan in hopes of softening the hostility of the medical profession. What had begun in the 1930s as a movement to redistribute medical services for the entire population turned into a proposal to help defray some of the hospital costs of social security pensioners.

THE APPEAL OF FOCUSING ON THE AGED

The selection of the aged as the problem group is comprehensible in the context of American politics, however distinctive it appears in comparative perspective. Unlike America, no other industrial country in the world has begun its government health insurance program with the aged. The typical pattern has been the initial coverage of low-income workers, with subsequent extensions to dependents and then to higher-income groups. Insuring low-income workers, however, involves use of means tests, and the cardinal assumption of social security advocates in America has been that the stigma of such tests must be avoided. In having to avoid both general insurance and humiliating means tests, the Federal Security Agency strategists were left with finding a socio-economic group whose average member could be presumed to be in need. The aged passed this test easily; everyone intuitively knew the aged were worst off. Cohen was later to say that the subsequent massing of statistical data to prove the aged were sicker, poorer, and less insured than other adult groups was like using a steamroller to crush an ant of opposition.

Everyone also knew that the aged—like children and the disabled—commanded public sympathy. They were one of the few population groupings about whom one could not say the members should take care of their financial-medical problems by earning and saving more money. The American social security system makes unemployment (except for limited part-time work) a condition for the receipt of pensions, and a fixed retirement age is widely accepted as desirable public policy. In addition, the postwar growth in private health insurance was uneven, with lower proportions of the aged covered, and the extent of their insurance protection more limited than that enjoyed by the working population (HEW, 1964, 22). Only the most contorted reasoning could blame the aged for this condition by attributing their insurance status to improvidence. Retirement forces many workers to give up work-related group insurance. The aged could not easily shift to individual policies because they comprised a high-risk group, which insurance companies were reluctant to cover except at relatively expensive premium rates. The alternative of private insurance seemed in the 1950s incapable of coping with the stubborn fact that the aged were subject to inadequate private coverage at a time when their medical requirements were greatest and their financial resources were lowest.

Under these circumstances many of the aged fell back upon their children for financial assistance, thus giving the Medicare emphasis upon the aged additional political appeal. The strategists expected support from families burdened by the requirement, moral or legal, to assume the medical debts of their aged relatives. By concentrating on the aged, the Ewing group believed they could gradually amass widespread sympathy for their plan, leading to a broad agreement that the problem they had defined could be solved by nothing less than congressional action on their proposed Medicare solution.

The same strategy of seeking broad public agreement was evident in the benefits and financial arrangements chosen. The 1951 selection of hospitalization benefits reflected the search for a "problem" less disputable than the one to which the Truman plans had been addressed. General health insurance was a means for solving the problem of the unequal distribution of medical care services; its aim was to make health care more equally accessible by removing financial barriers to utilizing those services, an aim broadly similar to that of the British National Health Service. A program of hospital insurance identifies the aged's problem not as the inaccessibility of health services, but the *financial consequences of using those services*. The provision of 60 days of free hospital care only indirectly encourages preventive health measures and cannot allay financial problems of the long-term chronically ill. The hospital benefit was designed, however, not so much to cope

with all the health problems of the elderly as to reduce their most onerous financial difficulties. Ewing and his advisers were well aware that
this shift in emphasis left gaping inadequacies. But, in the context of
the early 1950s, they took for granted that broader conceptions of the
aged's health problems were less susceptible to political solution.

The differences between making health services more accessible and
coping with the financial consequences of hospital utilization were continually revealed in the next 15 years. The statistical profiles of the
aged—first provided by the Truman health commission of 1952—uni-
formly supported the popular conception of the aged American as
sicker, poorer, and less insured than his compatriots (Feingold, 1966;
Anderson, 1968; Greenfield, 1966). Health surveys reported that persons 65 and over were twice as likely as those under 65 to be chronically ill, and were hospitalized twice as long. In 1957–58, the average
medical expenses per aged person were $177, more than twice the $86
average reported for persons under 65 (Figure 1.1). As age increases,
income decreases, producing an inverse relationship between medical
expenses and personal income. In 1960, it was estimated that approximately "25 percent of the low-income persons in the nation are aged"
(Cohen, 1960, 5). While slightly more than half the persons over 65 had
some type of health insurance in 1962, only 38 percent of the aged no
longer working had any insurance at all. Moreover, the less healthy the
aged considered themselves, the less likely they were to have insurance; 37 percent of those in "poor health" as opposed to 67 percent who
evaluated their health as "good" had health insurance (Greenfield,
1966). Of those insured aged, a survey of hospital patients reported,
only 1/14 of their total costs of illness was met through insurance.
There could be no question that the aged faced serious problems coping
with health expenses, though it was easy to point out that averages
conceal the variation in illness and expenditures *among* the aged.

For those who saw Medicare as prevention against financial catastrophe, the vital question was which bills were the largest for any spell
of serious illness. The ready answer was hospital care. Not only was the
price of hospital care doubling in the decade 1951–61, but the aged
found themselves in hospital beds far more often than younger Americans. One in six aged persons entered a hospital in a given year, and
they stayed in hospitals twice as long as those under 65, facing an average daily charge per patient bed in 1961 of $35. Hospitalization insur-
ance was, according to this information, a necessity that the aged had
to have to avoid financial catastrophe. But what the advocates did not
point out was that financial catastrophe could easily overtake 60 days
of hospital insurance. Such a catastrophe is defined by the gap between
medical bills and available resources. Medicare's protection against the

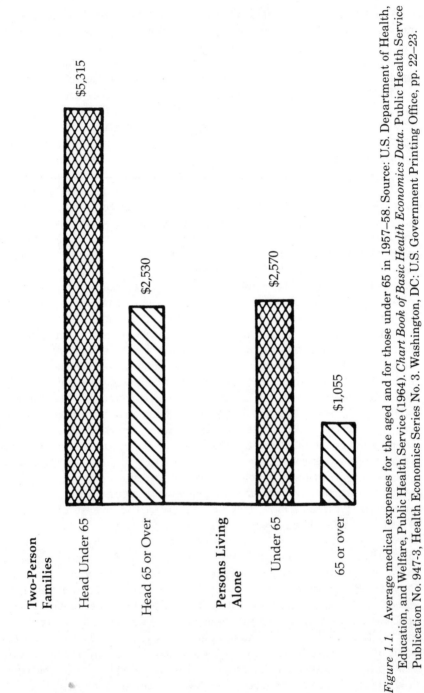

Figure 1.1. Average medical expenses for the aged and for those under 65 in 1957–58. Source: U.S. Department of Health, Education, and Welfare, Public Health Service (1964). *Chart Book of Basic Health Economics Data.* Public Health Service Publication No. 947-3, Health Economics Series No. 3. Washington, DC: U.S. Government Printing Office, pp. 22–23.

high unit costs of hospital care drew attention away from the financial costs of unusually extensive utilization of health services, whether high or low in average prices.

The concentration on the burdens of the aged was a ploy for sympathy. The disavowal of aims to change fundamentally the American medical system was a sop to AMA fears, and the exclusion of physician services benefits was a response to past AMA hysteria. The focus on the financial burdens of receiving hospital care took as given the existing structure of the private medical care world, and stressed the issue of spreading the costs of using available services within that world. The organization of health care, with its inefficiencies and resistance to cost-reduction, was a fundamental but politically sensitive problem that consensus-minded reformers wanted to avoid when they opted for 60 days of hospitalization insurance for the aged in 1951 as a promising "small" beginning.

FOCUSING ON SOCIAL SECURITY CONTRIBUTORS

The financing of the Truman health program had deliberately been left vague by its backers; the Murray-Wagner-Dingell bill of 1949 mentioned a 3 percent payroll tax, equally divided between worker and employer, and administered by a new division within the Federal Security Agency. In the 1951 promotion of a Medicare program, firm emphasis was placed on financing hospital insurance through the already established Old Age and Survivors Insurance system (OASI), enacted as part of the Social Security law in 1935. The use of social security funding was an obvious effort to tap the widespread legitimacy that OASI programs enjoyed among all classes of Americans. But it was a tactic with an equally obvious defect. Proof that the aged were the most needy was based on calculation for *all* persons over 65. Yet social security financing would in 1952 have restricted Medicare benefits to 7 million pensioners out of the 12.5 million persons over 65. This would have meant not insuring 5.5 million aged whose medical and financial circumstances had been used to establish the "need" for a Medicare program in the first place. Nonetheless, social security financing offered so many other advantages that its advocates were prepared to live with this gap between the problem posed and the remedy offered.

The notion that social security recipients pay for their benefits is one traditional American response to the charge that government assistance programs are "give-aways," which undermine the willingness of individuals to save and take care of their own problems. The Ewing group thought they had to quash that charge if they were both to gain mass public support and to shield the aged from the indignity of a means test. The contributory requirement of social security—the limitation of benefits to those having paid social security taxes—gives the system a resemblance to private insurance. Thus social security members would appear to have paid for hospital insurance. In fact, social security beneficiaries are entitled to pensions exceeding those which, in a strict actuarial sense, they have "earned" through contributions. But this is a point generally lost in the avalanche of words about how contributions, as a commissioner of Social Security, Robert Ball, once remarked, "give American workers the *feeling* they have earned their benefits" (Ball, 1964, 232). The notion that contributions confer rights analogous to those which premiums entail within private insurance was one that deeply permeated the advocacy of Medicare.

The public legitimacy surrounding the social security program made it an ideal mechanism for avoiding the stigma attached to most public welfare programs. The distinction between public assistance for the poor and social security rights for contributors is, in fact, less clear in law, and welfare legislation—for any class of persons—confers rights in this sense. But those who insist on the distinction between public assistance and social security focus less on the legal basis of rights than on the different ways in which these programs are viewed and administered. Social security manuals insist on treating beneficiaries as "claimants," and stress that the government "owes" claimants their benefits. The stereotype of welfare is comprised of legacies from charity and the notorious Poor Laws, a combination of unappealing associations connected with intrusive investigation of need, invasion of privacy, and loss of citizenship rights. The unfavorable stereotype of welfare programs thus supports the contention that social security funds are the proper financing instrument for providing benefits while safeguarding self-respect.

Ewing and his aides were concerned about securing the support of governmental elites as well as organized interest groups and the electorate. They proposed social security financing partly because of the political advantages it offered a president sympathetic to health insurance, but concerned about levels of administrative spending. Social security programs were financed out of separate trust funds that were not categorized as executive expenditures; the billions of dollars spent by the Social Security Administration were until 1967 not included in the annual budget the president presented to Congress, a political advantage not likely to be lost on Democratic presidents worried about the perennial charge of reckless federal spending.

These structural features of the politics of social welfare in America largely account for the type of "incremental" health insurance strategy adopted at the end of the Truman administration. They help to explain why the postwar Truman plans of comprehensive government health insurance gave way to a proposal to help defray some of the hospital costs of Americans over 65 who participated in the social security system. Massive public concurrence on the problems of the aged and the propriety of social security was an essential step in the strategy of the incrementalists. Hospital insurance for the aged would have to pass fiscal committees in the Congress, where the combined forces of southern Democrats and conservative Republicans were dominant. The difficulty of extracting social legislation from powerful, independent committees was a lesson that anyone involved in the Truman health insurance efforts could not forget. The strategy of the incrementalists after 1952 was consensus-mongering: the identification of less disputed problems and the advocacy of modest solutions that ideological conservatives would have difficulty in attacking. "In the beginning," recalled Wilbur Cohen, one of the coauthors of the first Medicare bill, "we looked at [the bill in 1952] as a small way of starting something big" (Harris, 1966, 55). The incrementalists, however small their initial demands, were not able to avoid a full, public battle over their proposals once the Congress, in 1958, was moved to hold hearings before the Ways and Means Committee on hospital insurance for the aged.

PRESSURE GROUPS AND MEDICARE: THE LOBBYING OF MILLIONS

Serious congressional interest in special health insurance programs for the aged developed in 1958, six years after the initial Medicare proposal. From 1958 to 1965, the congressional finance committees held annual hearings, which became a battleground for hundreds of pressure groups. The same intemperate debate of the Truman years (and often the same debaters) reappeared. The acrimonious discussion of the problems, prospects, and desires of the aged illustrated a lesson of the Truman period: the federal government's role in the financing of personal health services is one of the small class of public issues that can be counted on to activate deep, emotional, and bitter cleavages between what political commentators call "liberal" and "conservative" pressure groups. In the press, commentators felt compelled to write blow-by-blow descriptions of pressure group harangues and congressional responses. Within the Congress, clusters of Republicans and conservative southern Democrats allied to oppose "government medicine" and to declare war against this "entering wedge of the Socialized State." The president of the AMA captured the mood of Medicare's critics in testifying before the Ways and Means Committee in 1963; hospital insurance for the aged, he said, was not "only unnecessary, but also dangerous to the basic principles underlying our American system of medical care" (AMA, 1963, 17).

For all the important differences in scope and content between the Truman general health program and the Medicare proposals, the lineup of proponents and opponents was strikingly similar. Among the supporters, organized labor was the most powerful single source of pressure. Organizations of the aged were the result more than the cause of these heightened Medicare demands. The National Council of Senior Citizens, formed in 1961 with AFL-CIO financial support, claimed by 1962 a membership of 600,000 (Rose, 1967, 422). The AMA sparked the opposition and framed its objections in such a way that disparate groups only tenuously involved with medical care or the aged could rally around their leadership. Table 1.1, a small sample, representing a fraction of all groups involved in the lobbying, illustrates the continuity between the broad economic and ideological divisions of the Truman fight and that over health insurance for the aged (U.S. Congress, 1961a).

Three features of this pressure group alignment merit mention. First, the adversaries who are "liberal" and "conservative" on that issue are similarly aligned on other controversial social policies like federal aid to education and disability insurance. Second, the extreme ideological polarization promoted by these groups has remained markedly stable despite significant changes in the actual objects in dispute, such as the much narrower scope of health insurance proposals since 1952. Proposals for incremental change in a disputed social policy typically fail to avoid disagreement about "first principles." The polarization of pressure groups on Medicare illustrated the typical structure of conflict

Table 1.1. Alignment of Groups for and against Medicare

For	*Against*
AFL-CIO	American Medical Association
American Nurses Association	American Hospital Association
Council of Jewish Federations & Welfare Funds	Life Insurance Association of America
American Association of Retired Workers	National Association of Manufacturers
National Association of Social Workers	National Association of Blue Shield Plans
National Farmers Union	American Farm Bureau Federation
The Socialist Party	The Chamber of Commerce
American Geriatrics Society	The American Legion

over "redistributive"[4] issues in America; the sides, in tone and composition, resembled the contestants in an economic class conflict and
framed issues in what Lowi (1964, 707) calls the terms of "class war."
Finally, public dispute continued to be dominated by the AFL-CIO and
the AMA, lobbying organizations capable of expending millions in the
effort to shape the scope of debate and to influence legislative results.
Since the 1940s these two chief adversaries have engaged in what the
New York Times characterized as a "slugging match," a contest of invec-
tive. Aaron Wildavsky's description of the conflict between public and
private power advocates in America is just as apt for the contestants
over Medicare:

> [They] have little use for one another. They distrust each other's motives;
> they question each other's integrity; they doubt each other's devotion to
> the national good. Each side expects the other to play dirty, and each can
> produce substantiating evidence from the long history of their dispute.
> (Wildavsky, 1962, 5–6)

The American Medical Association is an organization with conflicting
roles. As a type of professional trade union, it is committed to improving
the status of physicians. As a scientific organization, the AMA sponsors
research and regulates medical practice to improve the quality of health
care available to American consumers. As a pressure group, the AMA
has fused these roles, linking, and to some extent confusing the issues
on which physicians speak as scientific authorities and as self-interested professionals. Its broad lobbying aim has been to convince the
American public that physicians are the sole authority that can properly decide on the organization, financing, and regulation of medical
care practice. Its major tactic has been to frame the dispute over issues
like Medicare so that proponents of federal action meet the widest possible range of ideological objections. The AMA has rallied groups against
Medicare behind the slogans of freedom of choice, individualism, distaste for bureaucracy, and hatred of the welfare state, collectivism, and
higher taxes. Under such banners have trooped organizations distantly
related to health insurance legislation: professional organizations,
business and fraternal groups, farm organizations, and various right-
wing protest groups.

The mixture of trade unionism and professional activities in the
AMA has undermined the credibility of either role. Physicians enjoy
both high status and high income (over $34,000 median income after
expenses, according to 1964 data from *Medical Economics*). The image
of the tireless and selfless practitioner has enhanced the authority of
medical organizations in public discourse. Yet recent trends, accompa-

nying the lobbying activities of the AMA, have weakened the claims of medical doctors to disinterested community leadership. Increased specialization (and with that the gradual disappearance of the general practitioner), rising fees, the greater impersonality of medical practice in the modern hospital setting—all have contributed to public dissatisfaction with physicians. The persistent AMA involvement with public policy issues since World War II has increased the risks that an image of the rich and greedy physician will replace that of the noble general practitioner and thus undermine the widely accepted role of the AMA (and its local affiliates) as controllers of medical practice. In these areas, organizations like the AFL-CIO feel less tension; their straightforward championing of the interest of wage-earners means that opponents have little opportunity to dwell upon the gap between the pronouncements of selflessness and the practice of self-interested maneuvering.

Both the AFL-CIO and the AMA have the membership, resources, and experience to engage in multimillion-dollar lobbying. Their members are sufficiently spread geographically to make congressional electioneering relatively easy to organize. In 1965, the AMA had 159,000 dues-paying members, and expended a budget of approximately $23 million. The AFL-CIO's 120 affiliated unions represented in the mid-1960s over $34,000 median income 13 million workers; it managed to spend nearly $1 million in the 1964 elections (*Congressional Quarterly* 1965b, 77–78). Both organizations control legally separate political bodies that disseminate propaganda, try to influence elections, and mobilize members for political action. The AFL-CIO's Committee on Political Education (COPE) and the AMA's Political Action Committee (AMPAC; organized in 1961) both spend far more than they report as "lobbying" expenditures. Lobbying—personal contact between organization officials and members of the government[5]—keeps substantial full-time staffs busy in Washington, but the largest organizational expenditures are for what is euphemistically called "public education." In 1964, COPE's educational tasks cost almost $1 million (*Wall Street Journal,* February 8, 1965). In 1965, the AMA spent just under $1 million, of which $830,000 went for the newspaper, radio, and television campaign against the passage of the Medicare bill (*Congressional Quarterly* 1965c; personal interview with Ernest Howard, director of the AMA, 1965).

During the debates of the 1940s and early 1950s, the American Medical Association and its allies in big business and commercial agriculture found it a relatively successful tactic to focus the debate on the evils of collectivism and socialized medicine. The narrowing of health insurance proposals from universal coverage to the aged, however, set new constraints on the anti-Medicare campaigns. In response to the Medicare bills, the aged themselves began to organize into such pressure groups as the Senior Citizens' Councils and the Golden Ring Clubs. Although these groups suffered a lack of the financial and membership resources that characterized the better organized lobbies, it was far more difficult for the AMA to engage in open warfare with them than it had been for the doctors to do battle with the powerful AFL-CIO. When the critics of governmental Medicare proposals seized on broad ideological objections, they now had also to take into account the possibility of being labeled the enemy of America's senior citizens. One effect attributable to this set of circumstances was the appearance of a conservative willingness to offer alternatives. In the late 1940s, Republicans and their allies in the world of big business and organized medicine offered nothing but the status quo in opposition to the health insurance schemes of that period. By the 1950s, a change of tactics was in order: it was one thing to write off socialism, but the risks of writing off the aged would give the wise politician some second thoughts.

NOTES

1.   The Blue Cross Association comprises nonprofit hospital insurance organizations affiliated with the American Hospital Association and its state members; Blue Shield plans, sponsored by state medical societies, are nonprofit medical insurance organizations whose boards of directors have been composed mostly of physicians.

2.   The three key officials—Arthur Altmeyer, Wilbur Cohen, and I. S. Falk— worked in the Social Security Board, a division of the Federal Security Agency. The FSA, created in 1939 to oversee the board, the Public Health Service, and the Office of Education, was in 1953 replaced by the cabinet-rank Department of Health, Education and Welfare.

3.   Wilbur J. Cohen, who in 1965 was Under-Secretary of the Department of Health, Education and Welfare, became HEW secretary in March 1968. Cohen was a member of the staff of the original committee that drafted the Social Security Act of 1935. He was, in 1952, an adviser to Oscar Ewing, the Federal Security Agency head, as was I. S. Falk.

4.   By "redistributive" I mean policies that purport to change the distributions of benefits and burdens among broad socioeconomic groups.

5.   This restrictive definition of lobbying accounts for the discrepancy between what pressure groups report as lobbying expenses and what they spend in trying to influence public policy. U.S. law (the Federal Regulation of Lobbying Act, 1946) defines lobbying as personal contact between group representatives and officials and only requires that sums expended for that purpose be reported. Hence, the large expenditures for propaganda in the mass media go officially unrecorded.

2

The Politics of Legislative Impossibility

MEDICARE UNDER A REPUBLICAN PRESIDENT

A t no time during the Eisenhower Administrations (1953–60) did the Ewing Medicare bills have a chance of congressional enactment. Hospital insurance for the aged lacked the political sponsorship that makes controversial bills legislative possibilities. President Eisenhower had campaigned in 1952 against "socialized medicine," by which he meant both the Truman health plan and the more modest proposals for the aged. The absence of presidential sponsorship was compounded by congressional resistance in the tax committees responsible for social security bills (Ways and Means in the House, the Finance Committee in the Senate), where the members were in the main either uninterested or hostile. Among congressmen generally there was not an intensely committed majority disposed to force those committees to report health insurance legislation. Even when the Democrats regained control of the Congress in 1954, the partisan majority did not comprise a favorable Medicare majority. In fact, the legislative prospects were so slight that no committee hearings were held until 1958. "Compulsory health insurance for the general population," it was clear, "declined as a legislative issue in the 1950s" (Legislative Reference Service, 1963, 1).

The enthusiasm of Medicare's promoters for future action persisted despite the obstacles of the Eisenhower years. To hasten that future, a group of men who had played important roles in the Truman health insurance efforts pursued their strategy of gradualism. Annually from 1952 to 1960, modest Medicare bills were introduced in Congress, not with any hopes for enactment, but to keep alive the idea of health insurance under social security. At the same time, these promoters turned their energies toward other social reforms. Wilbur Cohen, for instance, director of research for the Social Security Administration until 1956, actively campaigned for disability insurance covering work-ers over the age of 50. He did so on the assumption that by slowly expanding the number of impoverishing conditions insured against by social security, the risk of catastrophic health expenses would be left as the obvious major omission within the social insurance program requiring remedial legislation.

Once disability insurance was enacted in 1956, the strategists of gradualism concentrated again on Medicare. The four most active members of this group included Cohen, in 1956 about to take up a pro-fessorship of welfare administration at the University of Michigan; I. S. Falk, then a consultant to the United Mine Workers; Nelson Cruik-shank, head of the AFL-CIO's Department of Social Security; and Robert Ball, a highly respected career official in the Social Security Administration. Their tactical plan was twofold: to prompt congres-sional interest in Medicare by persuading a well-placed congressman to sponsor the bill, and to elicit wide public concern about the health and finances of the aged through an AFL-CIO propaganda campaign.

The advocates were successful in both efforts. Although the three most senior members of the Ways and Means Committee rebuffed the Cohen group's entreaties to sponsor its bill, the fourth-ranking Demo-crat, Aime Forand, from Rhode Island, responded. In 1958, hearings were held on the Forand bill. Organized labor, which through most of the early 1950s had concentrated on securing health insurance for its mem-bers through collective bargaining (Munts, 1967), whipped up a cam-paign for Medicare in anticipation of the Forand hearings. The hearings prompted the AMA into action as well; it raised its 1958 lobbying budget fivefold, and spent a quarter of a million dollars criticizing the Forand bill. The propaganda battle of the 1940s resumed, with each side match-ing the other in press releases, speeches, pamphlets, and harangues. Inadvertently, the activity of the AMA assisted its opponents in direct-ing public attention toward health insurance for the aged. Congressman Forand put the point facetiously when he expressed his indebtedness to the "American Medical Association for publicizing my bill so well" (Harris, 1966, 83).

The reopening of extensive public debate did not mean the Forand bill had favorable congressional prospects. In 1959 the Ways and Means Committee rejected the proposal by a decisive margin, in a 17–8 vote. That defeat left many prolabor congressmen acutely dissatisfied, but their numbers in the last two years of the Eisenhower administra-tion were too small to force a reconsideration. Yet the aim of renewing interest in social security health insurance had been served. The pres-sure groups aligned themselves in the "liberal" and "conservative" camps of the Truman years, and turned to the mass media to transmit their continuing claims and criticisms. Future demands for Medicare legislation would be forthcoming—that much was clear at the time hearings were concluded in 1959 and the Forand bill rejected. The question was how the Congress would deal with those future demands.

THE FORAND BILL VS. THE WELFARE APPROACH

The debate over the Forand bill revealed a pattern of disagreement that would continue to limit the alternatives facing the Congress. Both the problems defined as warranting public action and the type of proffered solution remained relatively stable from the time of Medicare's first introduction in 1952. The information gathered on illness, income, insurance status, and health care utilization almost invariably fell into the simple categories of the aged and the non-aged. When Forand's critics attacked his bill, they, too, shared the common focus of attention on the aged. Their argument from the Truman days that all Americans are not poor enough to warrant compulsory government health insurance turned into the argument that not all the aged are poor. That there were substantial health and financial problems among the aged was no longer disputed by the late 1950s. But the extent of those problems amongst the aged and the means of remedy remained the controversial subjects provoking polarized positions.

The disagreement over the merits of the Forand bill illustrated the persistent divergent approaches to problems of social welfare in American politics. One, the so-called social insurance approach, seeks partial solutions to commonly recognized problems through a financing mechanism that is regressive in character. That is, equal rates of tax are paid by all contributors up to an earnings ceiling, with the result that lower income persons pay a larger proportion of their income in social security taxes than do higher-paid workers. It selects beneficiaries not through tests of destitution, but by tests of presumptive need: the orphaned, the widowed, the disabled and the retired are *presumed* to be in need of assistance. Contribution to the social security system thus entails automatic payments of benefits to all those who fall into recognized circumstances of risk, regardless of income.

The alternative approach is that of private and public charity, based on the assumption that most members of a society protect themselves against unfortunate contingencies through savings and insurance. The remaining needs are those of the improvident, the impoverished, and the unlucky, for which the appropriate remedies are private charity or, failing that, local, state, and sometimes federal "charity" programs. Levels of payments under these programs are determined individually, by measuring the gap between the financial resources and the needs of the applicant. And the means of financing the benefits are either, in the case of private charity, the largesse of the successful or, in the case of government welfare programs, the general revenues of the federal treasury and/or state funds. General revenue funding in principle provides a more progressive tax base than that of social security in that, under general revenue-taxing procedures, the higher the income the higher the tax that is levied. The social security approach relies upon federal action; the welfare view is that the resort to federal action is the least desirable alternative.

This ideological division revealed itself in the Forand controversy on a variety of issues, but particularly over the questions of who needed help, what aid the needy required, and which financing and administrative mechanisms were most appropriate to the remedy.

(1) On the question of who needed help, the Forand bill specified all the aged participating in the social security system irrespective of their present income. Statistical profiles of the aged that were mustered in support of social security coverage emphasized:

- the high proportion of low-income persons among the aged (U.S. Census data indicated that in 1958 about three-fifths of persons aged 65 and over had less than $1,000 in money income, while another one-fifth received $1,000–$2,000).
- the greater incidence of illness amongst the aged (one indication was the National Health Survey finding that the aged received approximately twice as much hospitalization as those under 65) (HEW, 1962, 22–32).
- the inadequacy of private insurance coverage in meeting the needs of the elderly (social security administrators claimed that 53.9 percent of the noninstitutionalized aged were without any form of hospital insurance in 1959, although it was admitted that coverage amongst this high risk group was increasing. Forand backers, however, stressed the shortcomings of private insurance in meeting the total medical costs of the policyholders) (U.S. Congress, 1965, 40–44).

The critics frequently contested these and similar statistics on the aged, but their main theme was the numbers of aged who enjoyed good health, secure incomes, and private health insurance policies. Conceding that widespread health and financial problems did exist amongst the elderly, advocates of a welfare approach argued that the Forand bill did not address itself exclusively or effectively to those "who really need help," the very poor among the aged.

(2) The problem to which Forand directed attention was the catastrophic effects of large hospital and surgical bills; hence his benefits were limited to those expenses associated with expensive hospitalization and in-hospital medical care. Welfare approach opponents emphasized the inadequacy of surgical-hospital insurance for those whose means had been exhausted and who required outpatient care and drugs. They stressed the need for comprehensive benefits for those aged who could not deal with health expenses through savings, private insurance, medical charity, or state and local assistance.

(3) On the question of administration and financing, the Forand bill called for a federal program financed by social security taxes, emphasizing the contributory nature of OASDI and the desirability of not forcing the elderly to submit to the humiliation of a means test. Many conservative critics, who conceded that federal funds might be necessary to assist the medically indigent aged, nonetheless argued that expansion of federal power was undesirable. A more palatable alternative, to their way of thinking, was to share the financing of any medical assistance program with the states, reserving to the latter the role of administration and of setting standards according to local needs.

Hence, the irony of the dispute: the Forand backers focusing on all social security beneficiaries among the aged, proposing *limited* hospital-surgical insurance for them, to be paid for by *regressive* social security taxes; the more conservative welfare advocates proposing *broader* benefits for a small class among the aged—the destitute—and arguing that *progressive* federal tax revenues should be used, with the administrative organization in the hands of state and local officials. What led liberals to support the Forand bill was a skepticism that a means-tested, state-administered assistance program would actually be utilized or implemented. Table 2.1 illustrates the major differences in approach.

KERR-MILLS BILL OF 1960

The welfare perspective on health and financial problems was reflected in three stages. An initial skepticism about the extent of the crisis among the aged subsequently gave way to hope that the substantial health costs of the aged could be coped with by the private insurance industry. Finally, there was a tactical acceptance of the need for federal action. The Kerr-Mills bill of 1960 reflected the conception of appropriate federal responses that conservative congressional leaders felt compelled to offer as a substitute for Medicare proposals. The beneficiaries would be limited to those in severe financial need, but the benefits were subject to few federal limits. Standards of need and ben-

Table 2.1. Differing Approaches to Health Care

	Forand Social Security Approach	Welfare Approach
Beneficiaries	Only the aged who were covered under social security	Anyone over 65 whose resources were insufficient to meet his medical expenses
Benefits	Hospitalization, nursing home, and in-hospital surgical insurance (Medicare bills introduced after 1959 specified hospitals and nursing home insurance only)	Comprehensive benefits for physicians' services, dental care, hospitalization, prescribed drugs, and nursing home care
Source of financing	Regressive social security taxes	Progressive federal income tax revenues, plus state matching funds
Administration and setting of standards	Uniform national standards administered by the Social Security Administration	Standards varying by state, administered by state and local officials

efits would be left to the various states, and the funding would be grants-in-aid, from general treasury funds, to state administrations that agreed to provide their share of the funds for "medical assistance to the aged." These were the characteristics of the bill that Senator Robert Kerr of Oklahoma and Representative Wilbur Mills of Arkansas offered as a substitute for the Forand bill. In 1960, that alternative was adopted by both tax committees of the Congress and ultimately passed as Public Law 86-778.[1]

The Kerr-Mills program was broad and generous in theory. The federal government would provide between 50 and 80 percent of the funds states used in medical assistance for the aged, with the higher percentages going to the poorer states. Such arrangements, in the opinion of the Senate Finance Committee, would "enable every state to improve and extend medical services to aged persons." The expectation was that the 2.4 million persons on old-age assistance and the estimated 10 million medically indigent would share in the program. Senator Pat McNamara (D., Mich.) was more prescient. "The blunt truth," he told the Senate in August 1960, "is that it would be the miracle of the century if all of the states—or even a sizeable number—would be in a position to provide the matching funds to make the program more than just a plan on paper." Three years later, McNamara's predictions were confirmed by a report of his special Senate Committee on Aging.[2] In 1963, 32 of the 50 states had programs in effect, and the provision of funds was widely disparate among the states. Five large industrial states—California, New York, Massachusetts, Michigan, and Pennsylvania—were receiving nearly 90 percent of the Kerr-Mills funds, and yet their aged populations represented only 32 percent of the total population over 65 (Greenfield, 1966).

These predictable outcomes did not preoccupy the promoters of medical assistance to the aged in 1960. Both Mills and Kerr were prepared to cope with the worst problem—the health costs of the very poor among the aged—as a way of avoiding Medicare programs in the future. Both were quick to point out that their program allowed for more generous benefits than alternative social security proposals. In a later interview with a national business magazine, Kerr insisted on this contrast:

> The Kerr-Mills program provides greater benefits to those over 65 who need those benefits. The benefits include doctors, surgeons, hospitalization, nurses and nursing care, medicines and drugs, dentists and dental benefits—even false teeth. Each state can provide what is needed by the people within the state. The . . . social security approach for aged care would provide mainly hospital and nursing home payments. (*Nation's Business,* 1962)

Few states were in fact to provide such broad benefits; by 1963, only four states were providing the full range of care allowed for in the Kerr-Mills bill, and most programs imposed strict limitations on the conditions for care and the extent of care (Greenfield, 1966; U.S. Congress, 1963). But the program satisfied both those who genuinely believed in the desirability of state rather than uniform national administration and those who hoped even an unsuccessful Kerr-Mills program would head off the demand for Medicare.

The AMA, though originally opposed to the Kerr-Mills bill, soon came to understand its political virtues. In 1961, President E. Vincent Askey, M.D., urged the states to "implement [the Kerr-Mills program] for the needy and near-needy" (Askey, 1961, 12). Many of the state medical societies did not join in Askey's enthusiasm, but the cause of the AMA's concern was clear. The election of John F. Kennedy, who had pledged to promote enactment of a compulsory health insurance law for aged social security beneficiaries, had returned Medicare proposals to the front pages of the nation's newspapers. In late 1960, Kennedy recalled Cohen to Washington to head a health task force asked to draft a Medicare bill for introduction in the first session of the 87th Congress. When a policy has presidential sponsorship and favorable reactions in public opinion polls, and the partisan alignments in the Congress are supportive of the president, the chances of legislative adoption improve. The election of 1960 thus marked a pronounced shift for Medicare from the politics of legislative impossibility characteristic of the previous eight years to the politics of possibility.

NOTES

1. Wilbur J. Cohen, a lifelong advocate of health insurance under social security, wrote much of what became the Kerr-Mills law. Experts like Cohen were so familiar with the localistic, means-test approach to social problems that Kerr and Mills, who both had had long experience with Cohen, rather naturally called him from the University of Michigan School of Public Health to help draft their bill.

2. McNamara's special committee was created in 1961 to "make a full and complete study [of] the problems of older people." It regarded the enactment of Medicare as the aged's most vital concern and was a central clearinghouse for pro-Medicare information in the Congress (Vinyard, 1972).

3

The Politics of Legislative Possibility

MEDICARE, 1961

Kennedy had labeled his platform the "New Frontier," and included within it a variety of proposals for domestic change, which he promised "would get this country moving again." As part of the New Frontier, he prominently included a hospital insurance program for the aged. Shortly after his inauguration as president, Kennedy fulfilled his campaign promise. On February 9, 1961, a presidential message to the Congress called for the extension of social security benefits for 14 million Americans over 65[1] to cover hospital and nursing home costs, but not, in contrast to the Forand bill, surgical expenses. These benefits were to be financed by a one-quarter of one percent increase in social security taxes.

The *New York Times* headlined the proposal and forecast a "stiff fight" over the Forand bill's successor. The narrowing of benefits was but one obvious indication that the president and his advisers were aware of the strong opposition to his bill and that they concurred with the strategy long used by Wilbur Cohen. That strategy, designed to modify congressional intractability, soft-pedaled the innovative character of the program in an attempt to widen agreement on the legitimacy of government involvement in health insurance. "The program," President Kennedy reiterated, "is not socialized medicine. . . . It is a program of prepayment for health costs with absolute freedom of choice guaranteed. Every person will choose his own doctor and hospital" (*New York Times*, February 10, 1961).

Senator Clinton Anderson of New Mexico and Representative Cecil King of California—high-ranking Democratic members of the Senate Finance Committee and the House Ways and Means Committee, respectively—simultaneously and enthusiastically introduced the president's bill the second week in February. Neither, however, was regarded as the preeminent Democrat on his committee, and presidents typically try to have controversial bills introduced by dominant figures like Senator Kerr or House Ways and Means Committee chairman Mills. The lesser prominence of Kennedy's sponsors, coupled with the fact that the Kerr-Mills program was in its first year of operation as an alternative to Medicare, left no one in doubt that Kerr and Mills would prove formidable obstacles to the president's Medicare hopes. The ideological composition of the tax committees provided additional basis for skepticism about likely enactment. That the skepticism was well-founded was illustrated by the way in which Ways and Means dealt with the King-Anderson bill.

THE OBSTACLE COURSE IN CONGRESS:
FIRST TRY WITH WAYS AND MEANS

Kennedy's Democratic majority in the Congress presaged no clear majority favorable to Medicare, and only a majority vote of the entire House could extract the bill from a hostile Ways and Means Committee. Legislative liaison officials within the Department of Health, Education and Welfare counted only 196 House members certain to vote for Medicare in 1961—23 votes short of a simple majority. Only an intensely committed majority would even consider the unusual tactic of discharging a bill from committee. The House decision on Medicare thus would rest with Ways and Means.

The composition, style, and leadership of that committee provided ample grounds for predicting Medicare's defeat at the first stage of the formal legislative process. The 17–8 defeat of the Forand bill in 1960 indicated the combined strength of the southern Democrats and conservative Republican bloc on the committee. Kennedy's Medicare strategists would have to confront this coalition: in 1961, 16 Ways and Means committeemen were known to oppose the bill, including Chairman Wilbur Mills (D., Ark.), whose influence within the committee was formidable. Under those circumstances, the Gallup poll findings that "two out of three persons interviewed would be in favor of increasing the social security tax to pay for old-age medical insurance" (*New York Herald Tribune,* June 9, 1961, p. 11) provided little comfort to President Kennedy. Four votes—either southern Democrats or northern Republicans—would have to change for the president to have a Medicare majority within the committee, and the prospects were not good.

The sharp limits on the president's ability to secure the necessary votes are evident in the geographical and ideological character of the House Committee on Ways and Means. Of the 25 committeemen, 15 were Democrats, eight of whom were from southern or border states. Among the Democrats, there was a clear ideological division between six of the southern members and the others. The *New Republic,* a liberal weekly committed to a much expanded social welfare role for the federal government, indicated this ideological-geographical convergence in its annual evaluation of congressional voting behavior (*New Republic,* 1961). On twelve roll-call votes during the first session of the 87th Congress (1961), the *New Republic* found nine of the Democrats in perfect agreement with the magazine's position. The six other Democrats—all from southern or border states—voted in accord with the magazine's position 60 percent of the time or less. Among the ten Republicans on the committee, seven were in disagreement with the magazine's position 100 percent of the time; the remaining three 75 percent of the time. The nonpartisan *Congressional Quarterly* studies bear out the *New Republic*'s characterization of a substantial partisan cleavage, with a swing group of six southern and border state Democrats. Although the *Congressional Quarterly* analyses of the 87th and 88th Congress found Ways and Means Democrats and Republicans to be "more liberal" and "less liberal," respectively, than their party colleagues in the House, the Democratic showing was traced to the nine generally urban, prolabor members on the committee. Thus, despite the high average support among the Democrats for "liberal" measures, the coalition of ten partisan Republicans and the six more conservative southern Democrats easily comprised a negative majority on bills expanding the social welfare role of the federal government (see Table 3.1).

The conservative coalition opposing Medicare in 1961 was not a happenstance, but a predictable result of the committee's process of recruitment. Democrats on Ways and Means enjoy a unique source of influence, since they also comprise their party's Committee on Com-

Table 3.1. The *New Republic* (1962) evaluation of Ways and Means Democrats, 87th Congress, First Session

100% average approval	60% approval or less
King (California)	Mills (Arkansas)
Karsten (Missouri)	Harrison (Virginia)
Burke (Massachusetts)	Herlong (Florida)
Keough (New York)	Frazier (Tennessee)
O'Brien (Illinois)	Ikard-Thompson (Texas)
Boggs (Louisiana)	Watts (Kentucky)
Machrowicz-Griffiths (Michigan)	
Green (Pennsylvania)	
Ullman (Oregon)	

mittees, the group that makes all Democratic committee assignments. By convention, however, when new Democratic members of the Ways and Means Committee are to be chosen, the Committee on Committees defers the choice to regional party caucuses. For example, during the first session of the 87th Congress, two Democratic openings on the committee occurred through resignation: Thaddeus Machrowicz of Michigan and Frank Ikard of Texas. Their successors illustrated the pattern of geographical continuity: Martha Griffiths of Michigan replaced Machrowicz and Clark Thompson of Texas replaced Ikard. The effect of this customary practice has been to freeze the existing geographical distribution favoring southern representation and thereby to inhibit additions to the urban, prolabor group among the Democrats.

The nine Democratic liberals in 1961 thus operated in a committee whose structure made their social policy commitments a minority view. Most Ways and Means members enjoy an independence that made it unlikely that the president and the party could effectively pressure them into changing their votes. Widely regarded as one of the most prestigious House committees, Ways and Means attracts senior and influential members. Members stay on this preeminent committee a long time, and are more likely than other representatives to feel insulated from external pressures. Among the 1961 Democrats, for example, Frazier, Mills, and Herlong had served continuously since the Truman administration and many of the southern Democrats, including chairman Mills, had run unopposed as often as opposed in their districts. In the 1960 congressional elections, when 21 fewer Democrats were returned to the House than in 1958, no Democratic incumbent of Ways and Means lost his seat. Not subject to sharply fluctuating membership, Ways and Means is thus a kind of old-timers' club within the House; its members are beyond the range of pressure from House and executive leaders that younger congressmen, particularly those who need party help with reelection, may face.

As a rule, the committee is far more responsive to the wishes of the House of Representatives than it is to other sources of pressure. When a bill that is before the Ways and Means Committee has a strong majority on the floor waiting to enact it, its members usually feel a responsibility to report it. When, however, a controversial bill faces a bitter and close floor fight, the House frequently depends on the committee to "save it from itself." This gives Ways and Means the option of not reporting the bill at all or if it chooses to report the measure, of writing partisan compromises into it first.

The success that chairman Mills had in satisfying the House of Representatives is reflected in the reception that Ways and Means bills had there. The bills reported by Ways and Means are generally voted on under a "closed rule," that is, no amendments are permitted, only limited debate, and acceptance or rejection. This convention gives the committee great discretionary power in deciding what to write into their reported bills. House members go along with the convention because many of them have neither the time nor the expertise to master the complex technical details involved in tax, trade, and social security bills and because they prefer to avoid the pressure from interest group lobbies that those bills generally elicit. Maintaining the closed-rule convention for Ways and Means bills does, however, constrain the committee to deal responsibly with legislative proposals. Thus, despite the deep partisan cleavages on the committee, Mills maintained a reputation for not allowing partisan considerations to interfere unduly with its collective judgment on the technical merits of bills it handled. When partisan conflict was unavoidable, Mills took pains to contain it by compromises that sought to prevent massive Republican or Democratic defections from the bill as it was reported from committee. The pride that Ways and Means members take in the regular House acceptance of their reported bills further ensures their cautious handling of controversial measures like Medicare (Manley, 1965).

THE SOUTHERN DEMOCRATS

The chairman of Ways and Means had a pivotal role in the fate of the 1961 Medicare legislation. In less than a year after his own bill, cosponsored with Senator Kerr, had become public law, Mills again faced hospital insurance proposals he had helped to defeat in the previous session and that threatened now to displace the Kerr-Mills program. At the same time, his influence within the Ways and Means Committee was such that, could he be persuaded to support Medicare, it was likely that he could carry the committee with him.

When it came to dealing with Mills over the King-Anderson bill of 1961, Kennedy was in a difficult position. Medicare was only one of several major items on the administration's agenda. The president had initiated trade and tax bills of high priority to his domestic program, and these also fell within the jurisdiction of Mills's committee. Since Mills had agreed to introduce these bills in the House, and his support was requisite to their enactment, Kennedy and the House party leaders were at a disadvantage in pressing demands on him to back Medicare as well.

Mills's position in 1961 was affected by an election threat back home. The 1960 census returns required that Arkansas lose two of its six congressional seats, and in the process of redistricting it appeared that Mills would have to oppose Dale Alford in the district that included the whole of Little Rock. Alford was one of the two most conservative and antiadministration of the Arkansas congressmen. A contest with him would have been the most serious Mills had faced in a House career dating back to the New Deal. It seemed reasonable to suppose that Mills would be disinclined to support legislation, such as Medicare, that in the minds of many Little Rock voters would be too closely associated with an excessive role for the federal government in social welfare policy.

In addition to the chairman, five other southern Democrats on Ways and Means were opposed to the King-Anderson bill. The president needed at least thirteen pro-Medicare votes to have the bill reported to the floor, and took for granted that none of the ten Republicans on the committee would defect from his party's position. Hence, four affirmative votes were required from among those southern and border state Democrats who had voted against the Forand bill in 1960.

The 1961 Congress strikingly illustrated a key difference between the legislative politics of America and those of a cabinet-parliamentary system like that of England. Party, executive, and legislative leadership in the United States is not, as in England, in the same hands, and the platform on which a president rides into office need not reflect the aims of many of his fellow partisans whose assistance is crucial in the committee and floor stage of the legislative process. Kennedy's prospects for changing the votes of the crucial Ways and Means Democrats hinged on the House Democratic leadership: the speaker, the party whip, the floor leader, and the relevant committee chairman, Mills. While speaker Rayburn was ready to support the president's Medicare proposal, he lacked formal means to enforce party discipline on recalcitrant Democrats.

Of the six Democratic opponents of Medicare, Burr Harrison of Virginia was the least likely candidate for persuasion: a conservative southerner, he was both fixed in his ways and immune from pressure. At the other extreme was John Watts of Kentucky. He was reportedly willing to be the thirteenth vote for the King-Anderson bill if twelve others could first be mustered; he faced enough antiadministration sentiment in Kentucky to make conspicuous support of President Kennedy a personal liability. Among the other possibilities were the chairman, already a publicly announced opponent, and Herlong, Frazier, and Ikard, all of whom were at least six-term veterans of the House and had conservative predilections. Yet, since they were old acquaintances of speaker Rayburn, they might have been expected to go along with him in the absence of special district concerns.

Unfortunately for the legislative fate of the Medicare bill, at the very time when all the resources and skills of the House leadership were needed, the speaker himself was in failing health. Majority floor leader McCormack increasingly took on many of the informal leadership functions that Rayburn in the past had exercised so skillfully. The Massachusetts Democrat, though thoroughly schooled in the norms and sentiments of House veterans, could not be expected to have Rayburn's influence, enjoying neither the speaker's office nor the immense personal popularity Rayburn, a Texan, had with southern Democrats of the Watts and Ikard type.

The absence of Rayburn's highly personal legislative management, coupled with the past reluctance of the six "swing" Democrats to support health insurance under social security, meant that chairman Mills's position was unlikely to be challenged within his committee. The *New York Times*'s Washington correspondent, Russell Baker, judged this correctly only days after the King-Anderson bill was introduced. "The president's medical program," reported Baker, "despised by many of his own party inside the House Ways and Means Committee, was in great trouble" (*New York Times,* February 19, 1961).

Earlier in the month, the *Times* had emphasized the equally important fact that Ways and Means faced a "heavy schedule of high priority legislation," with the controversial Medicare bill unlikely to be discussed in hearings until late in the session. The certain opposition of Mills and Harrison, and the probable opposition of the four remaining members of the conservative southern group, held out dim hopes for those late session hearings (*New York Times,* 11 February 1961). In the meantime, the problem facing the president was not only to secure these southern votes on medical care legislation, but to have this group follow party leadership on the foreign aid, depressed areas, tax, housing, and trade bills.

When, as with the King-Anderson bill of 1961, it appears that a committee will not report favorably on a presidential proposal, the president and his allies have alternative strategies. The question facing President Kennedy was whether anything could be gained by any of three possible offensive strategies.

Kennedy could concentrate his bargaining resources on medical care, taking the chance of alienating support on other high-priority bills. Since the outlook for Kennedy's trade and tax legislation was otherwise favorable, both the president and his advisers agreed it would be unwise to press the Ways and Means Committee too forcefully. Moreover, the Democratic margin in the House (263–174) did not assure passage of the King-Anderson bill even if it were somehow to get to a floor vote: 60 or more of those Democrats appeared unwilling to pass Medicare in 1961. Hence a determined bid for House action was rejected by the president.

The second possibility was to try bypassing the House of Representatives with a Medicare rider to another bill. A rider is a bill that is attached as an amendment to another bill that has already passed one house. In April 1961, an increasing number of reports suggested the administration was preparing for a move in that direction. Senator Javits (R., N.Y.) expressed "dismay at reports that the administration had decided to put off a request for Congressional action until next year," and argued that "nothing will happen unless the administration gives [Medicare] priority at this session" (*New York Times*, April 5, 1961). The support of liberal Republican senators, coupled with broader sponsorship of Medicare among some Democratic senators, led Senator Anderson, Medicare's cosponsor, to deny late in April that legislative efforts for the session had been abandoned. The proposal was to add a Medicare amendment to the House-approved social security bill then before the Senate Finance Committee.

The Senate Democratic leadership, however, saw strong arguments against the rider tactic. Even if the composite bill passed the Senate, it would be reviewed by a House-Senate conference committee, and Mills's bipartisan influence within his committee was sufficient to force a choice between the social security bill stripped of the Medicare amendment or no bill at all. Kennedy and his advisers discarded the rider alternative, for the time being, and press speculation faded out.

A third option for Kennedy, the one he was to choose, involved accepting the defeat of the bill for that year, but using it to attract public attention to his thwarted campaign pledge. Although he had rejected the use of arm-twisting tactics within the Congress, Kennedy hoped to put indirect pressure on legislators by going to the public with an educational campaign about the legislation denied him in 1961. Whatever its short-term effects, that strategy ultimately had prospects of beneficial consequence.

THE KENNEDY ADMINISTRATION VS. THE AMA

Even before the King-Anderson bill was introduced in February, representatives of the Kennedy administration had begun castigating the AMA for trying, as Wilbur Cohen said at a Washington conference on the aged, "to thwart the will of the majority of the people" by "methods of vilification and intimidation" (*New York Times,* January 5, 1961). Although clearly the most immediate threat to enactment was the bottleneck within the Ways and Means Committee, it was the AMA and its supporters who drew most of the administration's fire.

The American Medical Association offered, to be sure, a conspicuous target. Eschewing compromise, the AMA employed every propaganda tactic it had learned from the bitter battles of the Truman era. "The surest way to total defeat," cautioned Dr. Ernest Howard, the organization's assistant executive vice-president, "is to say that the AMA should

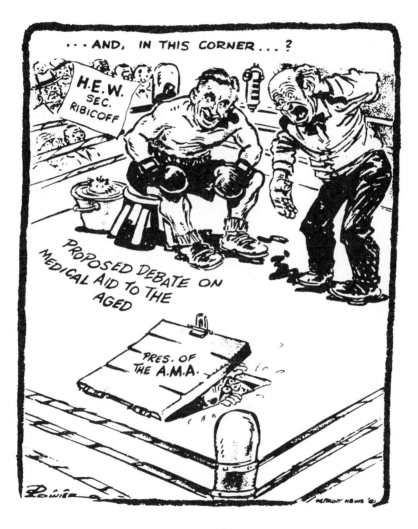

try to sit down and negotiate" (*Newsweek,* 8 May 1961, p. 103). Instead, AMA-sponsored newspaper advertisements and radio and television spots indicting the King-Anderson bill began appearing throughout the nation. Waving the red flag of socialism, these messages held out visions of a "new bureaucratic task force" entering "the privacy of the examination room," depriving American patients of the "freedom to choose their own doctor" and the doctor of the freedom "to treat his patients in an individual way."

The AMA simultaneously launched less publicized efforts to mobilize local communities against the Kennedy-supported bill. Congressional speeches criticizing H.R. 4222 were reproduced and distributed to newspapers and voluntary organizations. An "Operation Hometown" campaign began, enlisting county medical societies in a variety of lobbying tasks. The AMA equipped local medical leaders with a roster of ready-made speeches, reprints, pamphlets, sample news announcements, a "High School Debate Kit," radio tapes and scripts, and a list of guidelines for using the materials most effectively in teaching "every segment of the American public through every possible medium, [and stimulating] every voter to let his Congressman know that Medicare is really 'Fedicare'—a costly concoction of bureaucracy, bad medicine, and an unbalanced budget" (AMA, 1961).

As conspicuous as the AMA was in criticism, the administration's effort to confront the organization indicated the legislative frustration awaiting Medicare. Since King-Anderson supporters could do little to bring direct pressure on the pivotal congressmen in Ways and Means, they hoped their representation of the AMA as an unscrupulous and inordinately powerful interest that was successfully thwarting the public would cause congressional critics of Medicare to suffer guilt by association. In April, Health, Education and Welfare Secretary Abraham Ribicoff debated Senator Kenneth Keating (R., N.Y.) on television over the King-Anderson bill, and used the opportunity to lash out against the "scare tactics" of "organized medicine's" campaign against compulsory health insurance for the aged (*New York Times,* 5 April 1961).

The Ways and Means hearings of July and August provided another prominent occasion for continuing the bid for public support. The testimony of representatives from HEW linked the well-known case for the King- Anderson bill to a blistering attack on the pressure groups opposing it. The administration spokesmen, along with those of the AFL-CIO, diverted their attention from the specifications of the Medicare bill to the methods and interests of their medical, business, and hospital critics. The testimony of Secretary Ribicoff attempted to discredit AMA predictions of creeping socialism and the end of freedom by outlining again the modest character of Medicare. "The bill is designed," he said,

> only to take care of the aged. It is not my intention to advocate that we take care of the medical needs and hospital needs of our entire population, and the reason is that insurance is available for younger people. Blue Cross is available and it can be paid for by the working population. (U.S. Congress, 1961b)

Ribicoff stressed the two characteristics that most sharply distinguished English from American debates over government health activities. No hope was expressed of divorcing health care from consideration of finances, but only of taking care of a group with special problems in purchasing private insurance. Even the insurance was only to cover "unusual hospital needs," leaving out drugs, doctors' fees, and a whole range of other medical expenses. This raises the second point: the fact that the terms of the debate—the issues that proponents of the King-Anderson bill had to face—had been set by the opponents in the medical world. This pattern continued throughout the hearings, with the exception of the Socialist party's representative, who industriously tried to point out how modest and inadequate the proposed bill really was.

The press gave prominent coverage to the summer hearings, but the behavior of the committee members indicated that the bill's fate was a foregone conclusion. The southern Democrats, whose views were central to the committee outcome, were relatively quiet. Chairman Mills, who ordinarily took a dominant role in executive hearings on major bills, missed two of the nine open sessions, and remained dispassionate during most of those he chaired. Questioning was left primarily to a few of the anti-Medicare Republicans and pro-Medicare Democrats who were amenable to joining the propaganda battle being waged by those giving testimony.

At the end of nine days, on August 4, 1961, the hearings ended undramatically. A week later the *New York Times* reported that no further action on the King-Anderson bill was contemplated for that session. Amidst the national concern over Berlin and the call-up of reserve units, many Americans were unaware of the fate of what had been a campaign issue, or of the fact that Ways and Means had failed even to take a formal vote on the bill. Chairman Mills, unwilling as ever to highlight the partisan cleavages within the committee, and sharing with his fellow committeemen, and congressmen generally, a reluctance to clarify their public record with anything so concrete as a yes or no vote when there was little to be gained by it, preferred to let the bill die an anonymous death. If future events should force a reconsideration of the committee's position on Medicare—and Mills was aware of the possibility—a telltale 1961 vote might prove an embarrassment. Nor did the Kennedy administration, with an interest in future negotiations with Ways and Means, wish to burden Medicare with the legacy of a negative vote. The quietness of Medicare's burial made it easier for the bill's supporters to blame its murder on the AMA while diverting attention from the active complicity of the House committee and the passive complicity of the Kennedy administration.

Some analysts of American politics have confused Medicare defeats of the 1961 variety with AMA victories. "Measures apparently assured of passage," according to a *Yale Law Journal* study (Hyde et al., 1954, 995), "have been voted down, buried in committee, or substantially amended, upon the announcement of AMA disapproval." The AMA is thus pictured as a supreme legislative string-puller, the "only organization that could marshal 140 votes in Congress between sundown Friday night and noon Monday morning." Neglected in this stereotyped portrait is the distinction between results the AMA approves (or disapproves) and those they produce. The AMA has few resources for coercing individual congressmen to change their votes, especially senior, autonomous figures on committees like Ways and Means. That a coalition within the committee shared some of the AMA's ideological predispositions should not lead one to assume that the AMA controlled the votes.

This is not to say the efforts of pressure groups opposed to Medicare were unimportant, but rather that they were important in other ways. The AMA and its ideological allies brought the issue to public view in terms likely to place Medicare advocates on the defensive. Their impact was evident in the character of debate over medical care for the aged and especially in the narrowing of Medicare proposals to exclude coverage of physicians' care. But to account for the 1961 legislative outcome, one must turn from the public debate to the internal character of the Committee on Ways and Means. Only by doing so can one explain why the Medicare bill, initiated by the president and acceptable to a majority of Americans polled on the issue, could be undramatically defeated at the committee stage of the legislative process.

MEDICARE'S NEAR MISS, 1964

Between the defeat of President Kennedy's initial Medicare proposal in 1961 and the national elections of 1964, none of the major congressional obstacles to its enactment were fully removed. The Democrats maintained control of the Congress after the 1962 elections, but the proadministration bloc was, as usual, never as large as the number of

Democrats. In 1961, HEW's congressional liaison staff estimated the House Medicare breakdown as approximately 23 votes short of a 218 majority. The Ways and Means Committee never gave them the chance to check the accuracy of their estimates, and attempts to circumvent the committee with rider strategies proved abortive in 1962 and 1964. Each year hearings were held on Medicare, and by 1964, thirteen volumes of testimony had been compiled, totaling nearly 14,000 pages. But Wilbur Mills and his committee were not ready to report a Medicare bill.

The administration's pro-Medicare strategy included continued efforts to change votes on the committee. Two methods were employed. First, HEW officials were directed to respond to the objections of the key southern Democrats in hopes of bringing them around on the King-Anderson bill. When HEW assistant secretary Wilbur Cohen was informed of President Kennedy's assassination on November 22, 1963, he was in the midst of preparing changes in the administration bill that would answer some of Mills's criticisms. Cohen and his staff spent far more time courting critics than they did working with pro-Medicare members of the committee. The administration, through the influence of House Democratic leadership over members of the regional caucuses, also took steps to enlarge the size of the pro-Medicare group. After 1961, no new member of the committee was elected who had failed to assure the House leadership that he would vote for Medicare or, at the very least, would support its being reported out of the Ways and Means Committee. By 1964, these efforts had brought the total of pro-Medicare Democrats to 12, one short of a committee majority. Three of the anti-Medicare southern Democrats of 1961, Frazier, Harrison and Ikard had been replaced by fellow southerners who were willing to support the King-Anderson bill, Richard Fulton, Pat Jennings, and Clark Thompson, the latter the most reluctant. All the other Democratic newcomers between 1961 and 1964 were, like their predecessors, firm administration supporters.

This weakening of the anti-Medicare coalition revealed both the opportunities and risks that the politics of legislative possibility entail for Democratic reformers. Sensing victory within the Senate and realizing the narrow margin enjoyed by Medicare opponents within Ways and Means, President Johnson and congressional leaders thought again of a rider amendment in the Senate. But Ways and Means opponents were equally aware of the changed probabilities and nearly pulled off a clever legislative coup in the early summer of 1964. The senior Republican, John W. Byrnes of Wisconsin, proposed that the 5 percent increase in social security benefits that the committee had approved in earlier deliberations be increased to 6 percent. This would have raised social security taxes to 10 percent, widely accepted within

Congress at that time as the upper social insurance tax limit, and thus leave no fiscal room for Medicare in the future. The pro- Medicare committeemen realized the trap, but only 11 of their number were at the roll call vote. The anti-Medicare group seemed to have a winning margin, 12–11. But the final vote cast was by Bruce Alger, an archconservative Republican from Dallas. Unwilling to play the game, Alger voted with the Democratic majority, explaining later that "since he opposed the entire Social Security system, consistency would not permit him to expand it," even to undermine the chances of Medicare (Harris, 1966, 164).

Having observed their House brethren come close to catastrophe, Senate Democrats acted to attach the Medicare rider to the social security bill, which the House had already passed in 1964. But Mills had anticipated that move and, fearing that Ways and Means would lose control over the content of any Medicare bill, had taken steps to thwart it. He promised pro-Medicare Democrats on his committee that Medicare would be the "first order of business" in 1965; in return he received their support in rejecting the rider in the conference committee. With the House and Senate Republican conferees already anxious to stop Medicare, Mills had enough votes to accomplish this task. On October 4, the conference announced its deadlock over the entire social security bill, thus postponing both the social security cash benefit increases and Medicare until the following year.

The circumstances of Medicare's defeat in the fall of 1964 illustrated how substantially the possibilities of enactment had increased since the first Kennedy effort in 1961. The Senate was on record favoring the King- Anderson bill and the key bottleneck of 1961, the Ways and Means Committee, was within one vote of a health insurance majority. Wilbur Mills's promises for 1965 evidenced the weakened position of the anti-Medicare coalition. In September and December of 1964, Mills suggested to audiences in Little Rock that a soundly financed Medicare bill would gain his support in the next session of the Congress. Having already stated that medical care insurance would be the first order of business for his committee the following January, Mills expressed his concerns about the discrepancies between popular conceptions of Medicare and the content of the King-Anderson proposals. "The public," Mills warned in his Little Rock speech of December 7, "must be under no illusion regarding the benefits [and must understand that] Medicare does not refer to doctor services' or general outpatient medical care" (Mills, 1964).

Mills's worry was not ill-founded. "Medicare," a term that originally referred to the comprehensive healthy program run for servicemen's families by the Defense Department, was a misleading slogan for the King-Anderson bill. "Hospicare" would have been a more appropriate epithet. Despite the accretion of support between 1961 and 1964, the King-Anderson bills had changed only slightly. After 1963, Medicare was altered to include non–social security beneficiaries for a limited period, and here and there changes were made in the level of benefits. But the bill over which the conference committee deadlocked in 1964 remained basically a hospital insurance measure. When the deadlock was announced, observers, taking their cue from Mills's promises, assumed the King-Anderson proposal would be close to passage in 1965. In the meantime, the election of November, 1964, changed practically every political consideration; and Mills's ruminations in December about the unrealistic conception Americans held of Medicare was the first sign that anyone read the striking electoral victory of the Democrats to mean anything more than speedy enactment of a bill providing hospitalization and nursing home insurance for the aged. The *Congressional Quarterly* (1965d) soberly observed that "some type of medical care program for the aged is expected to be enacted by Congress in 1965."

NOTE

1.   The 14 million figure was an estimate for 1963, the first full year in which the Kennedy Medicare program could have operated. The projection of 14 million social security beneficiaries, out of a total aged population of 17.75 million in 1963, left an estimated 3.75 million aged uncovered by the Kennedy proposal. The proportion of the aged ineligible for social insurance benefits had been sharply declining since the original Medicare bill. Between 1950 and 1960 the number of aged receiving social insurance benefits more than quadrupled, from 2.7 million to 11.6 million.

4

The Politics of Legislative Certainty

THE IMPACT OF THE ELECTION OF 1964

The electoral outcome of 1964 guaranteed the passage of legislation on medical care for the aged. Not one of the obstacles to Medicare was left standing. In the House, the Democrats gained 32 new seats, giving them a more than two-to-one ratio for the first time since the heyday of the New Deal. In addition, President Johnson's dramatic victory over Goldwater could be read as a popular mandate for Medicare. The president had campaigned on the promise of social reforms—most prominently Medicare and federal aid to education—and the public seemed to have rejected decisively Goldwater's alternatives of state, local, and private initiative.

Within the Congress, immediate action was taken to prevent the use of delaying tactics previously employed against both federal aid to education and medical care bills. Liberal Democratic members changed the House rules so as to reduce the power of Republican-Southern Democratic coalitions on committees to delay legislative proposals. The 21-day rule was reinstated, making it possible to dislodge bills from the House Rules Committee after a maximum delay of three weeks.

At the same time changes affecting the Ways and Means Committee were made that reduced the likelihood of further efforts to delay Medicare legislation. The traditional ratio of three members of the majority party to two of the minority party was abandoned for a ratio reflecting the strength of the parties in the House as a whole (two-to-one). In 1965, that meant the composition of Ways and Means shifted from 15 Democrats and 10 Republicans to 17 Democrats and 8 Republicans, insuring a pro-Medicare majority. A legislative possibility until the election of 1964, the King-Anderson program had become a statutory certainty. The only question remaining was the precise form the health insurance legislation would take.

THE ADMINISTRATION'S PROPOSAL: H.R. 1 AND S. 1

Administration leaders assumed after the election that the Ways and Means Committee would report a bill similar to the one rejected by the conference in 1964. Hence Anderson and King introduced on January 4, 1965, in the Senate and House, respectively, the standard Medicare package: coverage of the aged, limited hospitalization and nursing home insurance benefits, and social security financing. The HEW staff prepared a background guide on the bill that continued to emphasize its modest aims. The guide included assurances that the bill's coverage of hospitalization benefits "left a substantial place for private insurance for nonbudgetable health costs, [particularly for] physicians' services." It described H.R. 1 as "Hospital Insurance for the Aged through Social Security," and no doubt would have encouraged the substitution of "Hospicare" for "Medicare" as its popular name, had this been still possible by 1965 (HEW 1965a).

Social security experts within HEW, with a rich history of sponsoring unsuccessful health insurance bills, were doubly cautious now that success seemed so near at hand. Wilbur Cohen, for instance, busied himself, with President Johnson's blessings, convincing the congressional leadership to give Medicare the numerical symbol of highest priority among the president's Great Society proposals: hence Medicare became H.R. 1 and S. 1. Its content, however, remained essentially unchanged. The HEW leaders, like everyone else, could read the newspapers and find criticisms that Medicare's benefits were insufficient, and that the aged mistakenly thought the bill covered physicians' services. The strategists believed, however, that broader benefits—such as coverage of physicians' care—could wait: the reformers' fundamental premise had always been that Medicare was only "a beginning," with increments of change set for the future.

The election of 1964 had a vastly different impact on critics of Medicare than on promoters of the administration bill, H.R. 1. If the election promoted satisfaction among H.R. 1's backers with their customary position, it provoked significant reactions among its opponents. Both Republican and AMA spokesmen shifted to discussions of what one AMA official, Dr. Ernest Howard, called "more positive programs." These alternatives grew out of the familiar criticisms that the King-Anderson bills had "inadequate" benefits, would be too costly, and made no distinction between the poor and wealthy among the aged. The AMA gave the slogan "Eldercare" to its bill, and had it introduced as H.R. 3737 by Thomas Curtis (R., Mo.) and A. Sydney Herlong (D., Fla.), both Ways and Means members. In comparing its bill and H.R. 1, the AMA earnestly stressed the disappointingly limited benefits of the latter:

Eldercare, implemented by the states would provide a wide spectrum of benefits, including physicians' care, surgical and drug costs, nursing home charges, diagnostic services, x-ray and laboratory fees and other services. Medicare's benefits would be far more limited, covering about one-quarter (25 percent) of the total yearly health care costs of the average person. . . . Medicare would *not* cover physicians' services or surgical charges. Neither would it cover drugs outside the hospital or nursing home, or x-ray or other laboratory services not connected with hospitalization. (AMA, 1965)

Claiming their "program offered more benefits for the elderly at less cost to the taxpayers," the AMA charged, as did some Republicans, that the public had been misled by the connotations of the "Medicare" epithet. Seventy-two percent of those questioned in an AMA-financed survey during the first two months of 1965 agreed that doctors' bills should be insured in a government health plan. Sixty-five percent of the respondents preferred a selective welfare program that would "pay an elderly person's medical bill only if he were in need of financial help" to a universal social security plan that would "pay the medical expenses of everyone over 65, regardless of their income." Armed with these figures, the AMA once again launched a full-scale assault on the King-Anderson bill, hoping to head it off with what amounted to an extension of the Kerr-Mills program.

By February, the issue was once again before the Ways and Means Committee. Pressure groups—medical, labor, hospital, and insurance organizations primarily—continued to make public appeals through the mass media and made certain their viewpoints were presented to the committee. Ways and Means had before it three legislative possibilities: the administration's H.R. 1, the AMA's Eldercare proposal, and a new bill sponsored by the senior Republican committee member, John Byrnes.

THE WAYS AND MEANS COMMITTEE AND THE HOUSE TAKE ACTION: JANUARY–APRIL

For more than a month Ways and Means worked on H.R. 1, calling witnesses, requesting detailed explanation of particular sections, and trying to estimate its costs and benefits. Executive sessions, closed to the press and one mark of serious legislative intent, began in January. The atmosphere was businesslike and deliberate; members assumed the administration bill would pass, perhaps with minor changes, and there was little disposition to argue the broad philosophical issues that had dominated hearings in the preceding decade. When spokesmen for the AMA invoked their fears of socialized medicine, they irritated committee members intent on working out practical matters, and chairman Mills refused to consult AMA representatives in further sessions of the committee's officially unreported deliberations.

Mills led his committee through practically every session of hearings on the administration bill, promising to take up the Byrnes bill (H.R. 4351) and the Eldercare bill in turn. By March 1, there had been continued reference to the exclusions and limits of the King-Anderson bill, with the charges of inadequacy coming mostly from the Republicans. On March 2, announcing his concern for finding "some degree of compromise [that] results in the majority of us being together," Mills invited Byrnes to explain his bill to the committee.

The Byrnes bill was ready for discussion because the Republicans on the committee, in the wake of the 1964 election, wanted to prevent the Democrats from taking exclusive credit for a Medicare law. The Republican staff counsel, William Quealy, had explained this point in a confidential memorandum in January, reminding the Republican committeemen that they had to "face political realities." Those realities included the certain passage of health insurance legislation that session and excluded the strategy of substituting an expanded Kerr-Mills program. "Regardless of the intrinsic merits of the Kerr-Mills program," Quealy (1965) wrote, "it has not been accepted as adequate . . . particularly by the aged, [and a] liberalization of it will not meet the political problem facing the Republicans in this Congress." That problem was the identification of Republicans with diehard AMA opposition to Medicare, which some Republican leaders thought contributed heavily to their 1964 electoral catastrophe. Hence Byrnes, who had been working since January on a Republican alternative, was anxious to distinguish his efforts from those of the AMA. At the same time, with the AMA spending nearly $900,000 to advertise its Eldercare plan, the criticism of H.R. 1's "inadequacies" was given wide circulation.

Byrnes emphasized that his bill, which proposed benefits similar to those offered in the Aetna Life Insurance Company's health plan for the federal government's employees, would cover the major risks overlooked by H.R. 1, particularly the costs of doctors' services and drugs. He also stressed the voluntary nature of his proposal; the aged would be free to join or not, and their share of the financing would be "scaled to the amounts of the participants' social security cash benefits," while the government's share would be drawn from general revenues (Cohen and Ball, 1965, 5). The discussion of the Byrnes bill was spirited and extended; the AMA's Eldercare alternative, not promoted vigorously by even its committee sponsors, was scarcely mentioned.

The Byrnes and King-Anderson bills were presented as mutually exclusive alternatives. HEW officials were exhausted from weeks of questioning and redrafting, and viewed the discussion of the Byrnes bill as a time for restful listening. But Mills, instead of posing a choice between the two bills, unexpectedly suggested a combination that involved extracting Byrnes's benefit plan from his financing proposal. On March 2, Mills turned to HEW's Wilbur Cohen and calmly asked whether such a "combination" were possible. Cohen was "stunned," and initially suspicious that the suggestion was a plot to kill the entire administration proposal. No mention had even been made of such innovations. Cohen had earlier argued for what he called a "three-layer cake" reform by Ways and Means: H.R. 1's hospital program first, private health insurance for physician's coverage, and an expanded Kerr-Mills program "underneath" for the indigent among the aged. Mills's announcement that the committee appeared to have "gotten to the point where it is possible to come up with a medi-elder-Byrnes bill" posed a surprise possibility for a different kind of combination. That night, in a memorandum to the president, Cohen reflected on Mills's "ingenious plan," explaining that a proposal that put "together in one bill features of all three of the major" alternatives before the committee would make Medicare "unassailable politically from any serious Republican attack" (Cohen, 1965). Convinced now that Mills's strategy was not destructive, Cohen was delighted that the Republican charges of inadequacy had been used by Mills to prompt the expansion of H.R. 1.

Byrnes himself was reluctant to approve the dissection of his proposal, humorously referring to his bill as "better-care." Nonetheless, from March 2 to March 23, when the committee finished its hearings, Ways and Means members concentrated on the combination of what had been mutually exclusive solutions to the health and financial problems of the elderly. Mills presided over this hectic process with confident but gracious assurance, asking questions persistently but encouraging from time to time comments from other members, especially from the senior Republican, Byrnes. The Byrnes benefit formula was slightly reduced; the payment for drugs used outside hospitals and nursing homes, for instance, was rejected on the grounds of unpredictable and potentially high costs. After some consideration of financing the separate physicians' insurance through social security, the committee adopted Byrnes' financing suggestion of individual premium payments by elderly beneficiaries, with the remainder drawn from general revenues. But while Byrnes had proposed that such premiums be scaled to social security benefits, the committee prescribed a uniform $3 per month contribution from each participant. The level of premium was itself a matter of extended discussion: HEW actuaries estimated medical insurance would cost about $5 per month, but Mills cautiously insisted that a $6 monthly payment would make certain that expenditures for medical benefits were balanced by contributions (*Congressional Report* 1965a, 61–62).

HEW was of course vitally interested in the uses to which Mills put the Byrnes plan. As one of the chief HEW participants, Irwin Wolkstein, explained:

Many features of the Byrnes Bill which had been objectionable were changed to be sure to keep administration support although some objections remained—including inadequate protection of beneficiaries against over-charging, absence of quality standards, and carrier responsibility for policy. The issue to the Department was whether the benefit advantages to the aged of SMI [Supplementary Medical Insurance] overweighed the deficiencies, and the answer of the administration was yes. (personal communication, December 11, 1968)

In its transformation into the "first layer" of the new "legislative cake," H.R. 1 was not radically altered. Levels of particular benefits were changed, reducing, among other things, the length of insured hospital care, and increasing the amount of the hospital deductible and coinsurance payment beneficiaries would have to pay. (Deductibles are the payments patients must make before their insurance takes over, and coinsurance contributions are the proportion of the remaining bill for which patients are responsible.) The continuing debate over these matters illustrated the divergent goals of those involved in reshaping Medicare. High deductibles but no limit on the number of insured hospital days were sought by those anxious to provide protection against chronic and catastrophic illness. Others insisted on coinsurance and deductibles so that patients would be given a stake in avoiding overuse of hospital facilities. But the most contested changes made in H.R. 1 involved the methods of paying hospital-based RAPP specialists (radiologists, anesthetists, pathologists, and physiatrists) and the level of increase in social security taxes required to pay for the hospitalization plan.

The Johnson administration recommended that the charges for services like radiology and anesthesiology be included in hospital bills unless existing hospital-specialist arrangements called for another form of payment. Mills, however, insisted that "no physician service, except those of interns and residents under approved teaching programs, would be paid" under H.R. 1, now Part A of the bill Mills had renumbered H.R. 6675. His provision required changes in the customary billing procedure of most hospitals, and became the subject of bitter disagreement. Such an arrangement, hospital officials quickly reminded the committee, would cause administrative difficulties and upset existing arrangements. But Mills stuck by his suggestion and easily won committee approval. More than any other issue, the method of paying these hospital specialists was to plague efforts in the Senate and conference committee to find a compromise version of the bill Mills steered through the Ways and Means Committee and the House.

Ways and Means also required more cautious financing of the hospital program than the administration suggested. Social Security taxes—and the wage base on which those taxes would be levied—were increased so as to accommodate even extraordinary increases in costs. The final committee report announced with some pride that their estimates of future hospital benefits reflected a "more conservative basis than recommended by the [1964 Social Security] Advisory Council and, in fact, more conservative than those used by the insurance industry in its estimates of proposals of this type" (*Congressional Report* 1965a, 54). [Mills's penchant for "actuarial soundness" was justified by Medicare's costs during the first year of operation; in 1966 both hospital and physician charges more than doubled their past average rate of yearly increase, thus substantially inflating program costs beyond HEW's initial predictions (HEW 1967a, 19, 31).]

Throughout March, Mills called on committee members, HEW officials, and interest group representatives to lend their aid in drafting a combination bill. The advice of the Blue Cross and American Hospital Associations was taken frequently on technical questions about hospital benefits. HEW spokesmen were asked to discuss many details with directly interested professional groups and report back their findings. Blood bank organizations, for instance, were consulted on whether Medicare's insurance of blood costs would hamper voluntary blood-giving drives. Their fear that it would prompted the committee to require that Medicare beneficiaries pay for or replace the first three pints of blood used during hospitalization. Throughout, Mills left no doubt that he was first among equals—he acted as the conciliator, the negotiator, the manager of the bill, always willing to praise others, but guiding the "marking up" of H.R. 6675 through persuasion, entreaty, authoritative expertise, and control of the agenda.

The Medicare bill the committee reported to the House on March 29, 1965, had assumed a form that no one had predicted in the postelection certainty that some type of social security health insurance was forthcoming. The new bill included parts of the administration bill, the Byrnes benefit package, and the AMA suggestion of an expanded Kerr-Mills program. These features were incorporated into two amendments to the Social Security Act: Title 18 and 19. Title 18's first section (Part A) included the hospital insurance program, the revised version of H.R.

1. Part B represented the modified Byrnes proposal of voluntary doctors' insurance. And Title 19 (now known as Medicaid) offered a liberalized Kerr-Mills program that, contrary to AMA intentions, was an addition to rather than a substitution for the other proposals. Essentially, the program provides for the unification of all medical vendor payments under state programs and uniform coverage for recipients. The provision in Title 19 that enables a state at its option to elect to cover individuals (regardless of age) not on public assistance, but whose incomes are close to the public assistance level, could also extend coverage to a significantly large portion of the poor population.

On the final vote of the committee, the Republicans held their ranks, and H.R. 6675 was reported out on a straight party vote of 17–8. When the House met on April 8 to vote on what had become known as the Mills bill, they gave the Ways and Means chairman a standing ovation. In a masterly explanation of the complicated measure (now 296 pages long), Mills demonstrated the thoroughness with which his committee had done its work. The health insurance program in H.R. 6675, Mills explained, was to cost about $3 billion. Byrnes presented his alternative bill after Mills had finished, and a vote was taken on whether to recommit H.R. 6675 in favor of the Republican alternative. The motion to recommit was defeated by 45 votes; 63 Democrats defected to the Republican measure, and only 10 Republicans voted with the Democratic majority. Once it was clear that H.R. 6675 would pass, party lines re-formed and the House sent the Mills bill to the Senate by an overwhelming margin of 315–115.

What had changed Mills from a Medicare obstructionist to an expansion-minded innovator? Critics speculated on whether the shift represented "rationality" or "rationalization," but none doubted Mills's central role in shaping the contents of the new legislative proposal. The puzzle includes two distinct issues: why did Mills seek to expand the administration's bill, and what explains the form of the expansion he helped to engineer?

By changing from opponent to manager, Mills assured himself control of the content of H.R. 1 at a time when it could have been pushed through the Congress despite him. By encouraging innovation, and incorporating more generous benefits into the legislation, Mills undercut claims that his committee had produced an "inadequate" bill. In both respects, Mills became what Tom Wicker of the *New York Times* termed the "architect of victory for medical care, rather than just another devoted but defeated supporter" of the Kerr-Mills welfare approach (*New York Times*, 1965). Mills's conception of himself as the active head of an autonomous, technically expert committee helps explain his interest in shaping legislation he could no longer block, and his preoccupation with cautious financing of the social security system made him willing to combine benefit and financing arrangements that had been presented as mutually exclusive alternatives. The use of general revenues and beneficiary premiums in the financing of physicians' service insurance made certain the aged and the federal treasury, not the social security trust funds, would have to finance any benefit changes. In an interview during the summer of 1965, Mills explained that inclusion of medical insurance would "build a fence around the Medicare program" and forestall subsequent demands for liberalization that "might be a burden on the economy and the social security program." What Mills may have meant, as one government official explained off-the-record, was that Ways and Means could avoid "physician coverage in the future under social security by providing it now under the [Supplementary Medical Insurance] approach."

In sharp contrast to Mills's flexibility, HEW cautiously had settled for proposing its familiar King-Anderson plan. In comparison with the committed Medicare advocates, Mills was the more astute in realizing how much the Johnson landslide of 1964 had changed the constraints and incentives facing the 89th Congress. President Johnson, busy with the demands of a massive set of executive proposals, was willing to settle for the hospitalization insurance that the election had guaranteed. Liberal supporters of the Johnson administration were astounded by the Ways and Means Committee's improvement of Medicare and befuddled by its causes. The *New Republic* (1965) captured the mood of this public at the time of the House vote, suggesting that the Mills bill could "only be discussed in superlatives":

> Fantastically enough, there was a tendency to expand [the administration's bill] in the House Committee. Republicans and the American Medical Association complained that Medicare "did not go far enough." Trying to kill the bill they offered an alternative—a voluntary insurance plan covering doctor's fees, drugs, and similar services. What did the House Ways and Means Committee do? It added [these features] to its own bill. Will this pass? We don't know, but some bill will pass.

H.R. 6675 PASSES THE SENATE: APRIL–JULY

There was really no doubt that the expansion of Medicare would be sustained by the more liberal Senate and its Finance Committee. But the precise levels of benefits and form of administration were by no means certain. The Finance Committee chairman, Russell Long (D., La.), held extended hearings during April and May, and the committee took nearly another month amending the House-passed bill in executive sessions. Two issues stood out in these discussions: whether to accept the payment method for in-hospital specialists on which Mills had insisted, and whether even more comprehensive benefits could be financed by varying the hospital deductible with the income of beneficiaries.

The first issue was taken up, with White House encouragement, by Senator Paul Douglas (D., Ill.). The question of specialist payment brought out in the open a dispute within the medical care industry. The American Hospital Association told the Finance Committee that encouraging hospital specialists to charge patients separately would both "tend to increase the overall cost of care to aged persons" and imperil the hospital as the "central institution in our health service system" (Feingold, 1966, 114). HEW's general counsel, Alanson Willcox, prepared a list of supporting arguments that Wilbur Cohen supplied in defense of the Douglas amendment to pay RAPP specialists as specified in the original H.R. 1. "These specialists," Willcox pointed out, "normally enjoy a monopoly of hospital business and yet they seek the 'status of independent practitioners' without the burden of competition to which other practitioners are subject" (HEW 1965b).

The AMA responded with fury to Douglas's revisions. Defending the specialists, the AMA hailed Mills's payment plan as a way to break down the "corporate practice of medicine" which made radiologists, anesthetics, pathologists, and physiatrists coerced "employees" of hospitals. "Medical care," the AMA told the Finance Committee, "is the responsibility of physicians, not hospitals" (Somers and Somers, 1967, 136). Apparently unconvinced, the Senators approved the Douglas amendment in early June.

In mid-June the Finance Committee approved a plan to eliminate time limits on the use of hospitals and nursing homes. The supporters of this amendment were a mixed lot of pro- and anti-Medicare Senators, and it was clear the latter group thought this change might deadlock the entire bill. For those who wanted more adequate protection against financial catastrophe there was the subsequent realization that a well-intentioned mistake had been made. With the White House and HEW insisting on a reconsideration, the committee scrapped the amendment on June 23 by a vote of 10–7. In its place, it provided "120 days of hospital care with $10 a day deductible after 60 days" (Irwin Wolkstein, personal communication, December 11, 1968).

The Finance Committee also took up a variety of provisions within the Mills bill that administration spokesmen considered "important defects." The Medicare sponsor in the Senate, Clinton Anderson, argued that paying physicians their "usual and customary fees" (the Byrnes suggestion) would "significantly and unnecessarily inflate the cost of the program to the tax-payer and to the aged." The House bill had left the determination of what was a "reasonable charge" to the insurance companies, which would act as intermediaries for the medical insurance program, and Anderson saw no reason why these companies would save the government from an "open-ended payment" scheme (Bray, 1965). Medical spokesmen, however, were so critical of the overall Medicare legislation that fears of a physicians' boycott persuaded Senate reformers not to raise further the sensitive topic of fee schedules for physicians.

The Senate, unlike the House at that time, does not vote on social security bills under a closed rule. This meant further amendments and debate would take place on the Senate floor on the Finance Committee's somewhat altered version of the Mills bill. On July 6, debate was opened and the Senate quickly agreed to accept the recommendation to insure unlimited hospital care with $10 coinsurance payments after 60 days. Three days later, after heated discussion, the Senate finished with its amendments, and passed its version of Medicare by a vote of 68–21. On the crucial but unsuccessful vote to exclude Part A from the insurance program, 18 Republicans and 8 southern Democrats took the losing side. According to newspaper estimates, the expanded bill passed by the Senate increased the "price tag" on Medicare by $900 million. The conference committee was certain to have a number of financial and administrative differences to work out through compromise.

MEDICARE COMES OUT OF THE CONFERENCE COMMITTEE: JULY 26, 1965

More than 500 differences were resolved in conference between the Senate and House versions of Medicare. Most of the changes were made through the standard bargaining methods of quid pro quo and splitting the difference. The most publicized decision was the rejection of the Douglas plan for paying RAPP specialists under the hospital insurance program. Mills's victory on this score was to cause much further alarm in the months to come, when the Social Security Administration began its administrative task of preparing for Medicare's initiation, July 1, 1966.

The bulk of the decisions were compromises between divergent benefit levels. The changes of duration and type of benefit involved either accepting one of the two congressional versions or combining different provisions. The decisions on the five basic benefits in the hospital plan aptly illustrate these patterns of accommodation:

1. *Benefit duration*—House provided 60 days of hospital care after a deductible of $40. Senate provided unlimited duration but with $10 co-insurance payments for each day in excess of 60. *Conference* provided 60 days with the $40 House deductible, and an additional 30 days with the Senate's $10 co-insurance provision.

2. *Posthospital extended care (skilled nursing home)*—House provided 20 days of such care with 2 additional days for each unused hospital day, but a maximum of 100 days. Senate provided 100 days but imposed a $5 a day co-insurance for each day in excess of 20. *Conference* adopted Senate version.

3. *Posthospital home-health visits*—House authorized 100 visits after hospitalization. Senate increased the number of visits to 175, and deleted requirements of hospitalization. *Conference* adopted House version.

4. *Outpatient diagnostic services*—House imposed a $20 deductible with this amount credited against an inpatient hospital deductible imposed at the same hospital within 20 days. Senate imposed a 20 percent co-insurance on such services, removed the credit against the inpatient hospital deductible but allowed a credit for the deductible as an incurred expense under the voluntary supplementary program (for deductible and reimbursement purposes). *Conference* adopted Senate version.

5. *Psychiatric facilities*—House provided for 60 days of hospital care with a 180-day lifetime limit in the voluntary supplementary program. Senate moved these services over into basic hospital insurance and increased the lifetime limit to 210 days. *Conference* accepted the Senate version but reduced the lifetime limit to 190 days. (*Congressional Report* 1965b, 4)

None of these compromises satisfied the pro-Medicare pressure groups, which had been anxious to make the law administratively less complicated. By late July, the conference committee had finished its report. On July 27, the House passed the revised bill by a margin of 307–116 and the Senate followed suit two days later with a 70–24 vote. On July 30, 1965, President Johnson signed the Medicare bill into Public Law 89-97, at the ceremony in Independence, Missouri, described at the beginning of this study.

THE OUTCOME OF 1965: EXPLANATION AND ISSUES

One of the most important lessons of Medicare's enactment is that the events surrounding its passage were atypical. The massive Democratic electoral victories in 1964 created a solid majority in Congress for the president's social welfare bills, including federal aid to education,

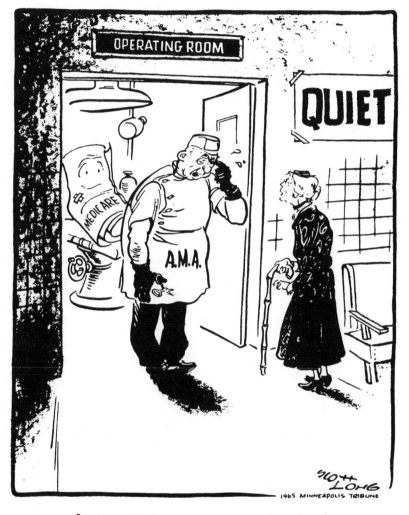

"THE OPERATION IS A FAILURE !...
THE PATIENT IS GOING TO LIVE !"

Medicare, and the doubling of the "war on poverty" effort. To find the most recent precedent, we must go back almost 30 years, to Franklin Roosevelt's New Deal Congresses. In the intervening years, we find a different pattern. Democratic majorities in the Congress have not been uncommon, but normally the partisan margins have been sufficiently close on many issues to give the balance of power to minority groups within the party. Under these circumstances, states' rights southern congressmen in coalition with Republicans have often been successful in blocking or delaying bills that entail the expansion of federal control.

The fragmentation of authority in the Congress compounds the opportunities for minorities to block legislation; bills must be subjected to committees, subcommittees, procedural formalities, and conference groups. To be sure, overwhelming majority support for a given bill can ensure that it will emerge, more or less intact, as law, even though it may pass under the jurisdiction of hostile congressmen in the process. However, it is extraordinarily difficult to create a congressional majority committed to an issue out of Democratic congressional partisans. President Kennedy, in 1961, avoided a major confrontation over Medicare because it was uncertain whether the bill could pass a House vote and because he needed the support of Ways and Means members for his other programs. Congressmen must frequently make similar decisions; for example, many representatives who supported Medicare before 1965 were nonetheless unwilling to launch a major drive to extract it from Ways and Means. Like the president, they often needed the support of Medicare opponents for other legislation that they believed was more important or had a better chance of successful enactment.

Within this context, backers of controversial legislation generally adopt a strategy that looks to the gradual accretion of support. They frame the issue so that opponents will find them difficult to attack, then set out to accumulate both mass public support and the necessary congressional votes. Particular attention is given to crucial committee bottlenecks. The executive relies heavily on the influence of the House and Senate leadership in this effort, and acts on the assumption that although it is seldom possible to change the mind of a congressman on the merits of an issue, it is sometimes possible to change his vote. While the congressional leaders lack formal means for enforcing party discipline, they have a variety of other resources. Their personal influence with the regional caucuses who selected Ways and Means committeemen, for example, allowed them to deny assignments to Medicare opponents and thereby to alter gradually the voting margin on the committee.

By 1964, the use of this accretionist strategy by Medicare supporters seemed on the verge of success; and had the elections of that year resulted in the usual relatively close partisan margins in the Congress, the Medicare Act of 1965 would have been much narrower in scope, and its passage would stand as a vindication of the incrementalist strategy. In fact, the 1964 elections returned a Congress in which many of the usual patterns of bargaining were less relevant. The Medicare bill that finally emerged as law must be analyzed in terms of the various responses to the highly unusual circumstances in that Congress.

In seeking answers as to why the legislative outcome differed so markedly from the administration's input, three separable issues are involved. Why did the traditional hospitalization insurance proposal pass as one part of the composite legislation? The congressional realignment after the elections of 1964 provides the ready answer. Why the legislation took the composite form it did is partly answerable in this way as well. The certainty that some Medicare bill would be enacted changed the incentives and disincentives facing former Medicare opponents. Suggesting a physicians' insurance alternative offered an opportunity for Republicans to cut their losses in the face of certain Democratic victory and to counteract public identification of Republican opposition with intransigent AMA hostility to Medicare. Wilbur Mills's motives are fully comprehensible only in the context of congressional conventions, especially the relationship of the Ways and Means Committee to the House, and the committee's tradition of restrained, consensual bargaining among its partisan blocs. However, if the political needs of the minority party and the Ways and Means members account for the Republican alternative bill and the committee's expansion of Medicare, the limits of that expansion require further explanation.

The context of the debate over government health insurance sharply delimited the range of alternatives open to innovators. That long debate—focused on the aged as the problem group, social security vs. general revenues as financing mechanisms, and partial vs. comprehensive benefits for either all the aged or only the very poor amongst the aged—structured the content of the innovations. The political circumstances of 1965 account for why innovation by Republicans and conservative Democrats was a sensible strategy. The character of more than a decade of dispute over health insurance programs for the aged explains the programmatic features of the combination that Wilbur Mills engineered, President Johnson took credit for, and the Republicans and American Medical Association inadvertently helped to ensure.

The outcome of 1965 was, to be sure, a model of unintended consequences. The final legislative package incorporated features that no one had fully foreseen, and aligned supporters and opponents in ways that surprised many of the leading actors. Yet the eleventh-hour expansion of Medicare should not draw one's attention away from the constricting parameters of change. Were a European to reflect upon this episode of social policymaking in America, his attention would be directed to the narrow range within which government health proposals operated. He would emphasize that no European nation restricted its health insurance programs to one age group; and he would point out that special health "assistance" programs, like that incorporated in Title 19, had been superseded in European countries for more than a generation. The European perspective is useful, if only to highlight those features of the 1965 Medicare legislation that were *not* changed.

Although the new law was broader than the King-Anderson bill in benefit structure, it did not provide payment for all medical expenses, P.L. 89-97 continued to reflect an "insurance" as opposed to a "prepayment" philosophy of medical-care financing. The former assumes that paying substantial portions of any insured cost is sufficient; the problem to which such a program addresses itself is avoidance of unbudgetable financial strain. The latter view seeks to separate financing from medical considerations. Its advocates are not satisfied with programs that pay 40 percent of the aged's expected medical expenses (one rough estimate of Medicare's effects); only full payment and the total removal of financial barriers to access to health services will satisfy them. In Medicare's range of deductibles, exclusions, and coinsurance provisions, the "insurance" approach was followed, illustrating the continuity between the first Ewing proposals in 1952 of 60 days of hospital care and the much-expanded benefits of the 1965 legislation.

Nor were major changes made in the group designated as beneficiaries under the insurance program. The administration had single-mindedly focused on the aged and the legislation provided that "every person who has attained the age of 65" was entitled to hospital benefits. Though this coverage represented an expansion over the limitation to social security eligibles in bills of the 1950s and early 1960s, the legislation provided that, by 1968, the beneficiaries under Part A would be narrowed again to include only social security participants. [This provision "applied only to persons first attaining age 65 in 1968 and after—only a very small fraction of the current aged—and the test of social security eligibility is less strict than is the test for cash benefits" (Irwin Wolkstein, personal communication, December 11, 1968).] The persistent efforts to provide Medicare benefits as a matter of "earned right" had prompted this focus on social security and, as a result, on the aged. While the social security system was not the only way to convey a sense of entitlement (payroll taxes in the Truman plans were included for the same purpose), the politics of more than a decade of incremental efforts had effectively undercut the broad coverage of the Truman proposals.

Title 19, establishing the medical assistance program popularly known as "Medicaid," made exception to the age restrictions. This bottom layer of the "legislative cake" authorized comprehensive coverage for all those, regardless of age, who qualified for public assistance and for those whose medical expenses threatened to produce future indigence. As in the Kerr-Mills bill that it succeeded, financing was to be shared by federal government general revenues and state funds. The Medicaid program, too, owed much to the past debates, growing as it did out of the welfare public assistance approach to social problems. Its attraction to the expansionists in 1965 did not rest on its charitable features alone. In the eyes of Wilbur Mills, it was yet another means of "building a fence" around Medicare, by undercutting future demands to expand the social security insurance program to cover all income groups.

The voluntary insurance scheme for physicians' services, Part B of Title 18, represented a return to the breadth of benefits suggested in the Truman plans (although, unlike the Truman proposals, it was neither compulsory nor available to all age groups). Since the adoption of an accretionist strategy in the wake of the Truman health insurance defeats, coverage of physicians' costs has been largely dropped from proposals. Throughout the 1950s reformers had focused on rising hospital costs and the role that the federal government should play in meeting those costs. Except for the Forand bills, proposals for health insurance between 1952 and 1964 fastidiously avoided the sensitive issue of covering doctors' care. Even when the election of 1964 eradicated the close congressional margin that had prompted the accretionist strategy in the first place, the administration continued to follow it. It was Wilbur Mills, and not the presidential advisers, who most fully appreciated the changed possibilities. Once again acting to build a fence around the program and insure against later expansion of the social security program to include physicians' coverage, he preempted the Byrnes proposal with a general revenue–individual contribution payment scheme.

For a decade and more, the American Medical Association had been able to dictate many of the terms of debate, particularly on physicians' coverage. And although the 1964 election revealed how much the alleged power of AMA opposition to block legislation depended on the makeup of Congress, the provisions for paying doctors under Part B of Medicare reflected the legislators' fears that the doctors would act on their repeated threats of noncooperation in implementing Medicare. To enlist the support of the medical profession, the law avoided prescribing a fee schedule for physicians, and directed instead that the doctors of Medicare patients be paid their "usual and customary fee," provided the fee was also "reasonable." Moreover, it was not required that the doctor directly charge the insurance company intermediaries who were to handle the government payments; he could bill the patient, who, after paying his debt, would be reimbursed by the insurance company. This left a doctor the option of charging the patient more than the government would be willing to reimburse. But congressional sympathy with the doctors' distaste for government control, and fear that doctors would elect not to treat Medicare patients under more restrictive fee schedules, made "reasonable charges" appear a sensible standard of payment.

The eligibility requirements, benefits, and financing of the Medicare program represent a complex political outcome, a mixture of continuity and surprise not typical of the legislative histories of other social welfare measures. The long process of building support for a hospitalization program covering the aged had not prepared the Johnson administration for the unpredictable opportunities of 1965. Instead of the King-Anderson bills of the 1960s, HEW had the Mills bill to turn into an operational Medicare program by July 1966. The politics of congressional bargaining had produced a considerably larger (and many felt a better) bill than the Johnson administration had proposed in the first weeks of 1965.

5

Medicare and the Analysis of Social Policy in American Politics

CASE STUDIES AND CUMULATIVE KNOWLEDGE

Case studies cannot by their nature prove anything. They can only illustrate the plausibility (or implausibility) of other conceptual, procedural, or substantive generalizations. This final chapter departs from the sequential organization of the earlier part of the book to explore the significance of the Medicare case and to attempt to set out some of these other evaluations. First, I discuss the underlying framework of analysis that guided the way I posed and tried to answer my inquiries. My interest in analytic frameworks arises from a concern that case studies be more cumulative than they have been. Only studies that employ comparable analytic models can be cumulated, and the first part of this chapter discusses both some representative analytic models and the use put to them in the bulk of the Medicare analysis.

Second, I compare the political processes and policy outcomes of Medicare with those of other issues to show how the processes that characterized the Medicare dispute are general to the redistributive arena of American politics. In policy content, Medicare exemplifies the social insurance model of welfare policy. Its beneficiaries, benefits, financing, and administrative structure conform strikingly to this pattern and are in equally striking contrast with those of public assistance programs.

Third, this concluding chapter addresses itself to some of the differences between legislative and administrative politics. The early implementation of Medicare illustrates the transformation of controversial, statutory proposals into operational programs that quickly become routinized, stripped of earlier ideological conflict, and beset by the competing and intense claims of groups materially concerned with their burdens and benefits.

CONCEPTUAL MODELS AND THE MEDICARE CASE

The discussion of Medicare politics earlier in this book was organized with self-conscious concern about how its conceptual structure could be adapted to cumulative policy analysis. This meant a continuing concern with how the problems of analysis were framed, what units of analysis were used, what focal concepts, and what patterns of inference. I want to make these underlying concerns explicit at this point and consider the explanatory effects of alternative analytic frameworks.

Conceptual frameworks give structure to the complex political universe for the analyst and in that sense are like lenses, that is, instruments that shape the field of vision, determine the level of detail, color the objects viewed, and limit the range of consideration. In reviewing the Medicare analysis from this standpoint, one is led to ask, What framework was implicit in its various parts, and what difference did it make in the analysis offered?

THE ORIGINS OF MEDICARE: THE RATIONAL ACTOR MODEL

In dealing with the origins of Medicare, the question was why government elites *chose* the early 1950s to narrow the focus of federal health insurance bills from the general population to the aged, and to restrict benefits to partial hospitalization coverage. Why, in short, did the Truman administration decide to adopt the Medicare strategy?

The unit of analysis used in the text was a strategic political decision. The explanation given for the strategic choice was in the form of a set of reasons why sensible men could agree on a new but less dramatic course of action. This type of explanation should be distinguished from an account of why the shift in strategy took place. Useless debate is furthered without care for such distinctions. The reasons men give for a course of action may differ widely from the fundamental causes for a course of action—in this case, a shift in political strategy.

The fate of the Truman health insurance proposals provided the immediate backdrop for strategic choice. The perception that the aged were more acceptable to the general public as a deserving group was the major reason they were the chosen target of concern. Likewise, the restriction of Medicare benefits to social security beneficiaries was explained by the observation that social insurance programs enjoy considerable legitimacy while public assistance programs that use the means test do not. The principal pattern of inference was to show what goals the reformers were pursuing in deciding to opt for the Medicare rather than the national health insurance strategy.

Thinking about a government as if it were a single rational actor is perhaps the most common analytic orientation of U.S. political scientists. The vocabulary of "choice," "purposive action," and "rational calculation" is so common in national policy studies that its users are not typically self-conscious about the assumptions on which their conceptual orientation depends. For many purposes, political occurrences may be properly characterized as the purposive acts of national governments, to summarize the varied activities of governmental representatives as the nation transforms "unwieldy complexity into manageable packages" (Allison, 1968, 1). But this productive shorthand has the capacity to obscure as well as aid; it does not take into account that what we call the government is in fact a loose congerie of large organizations and political bargainers.

According to the rational actor model, the happenings of national politics are "the choices of domestic actors." Policy is understood as the action of the rational decision-maker. The choices and actions of the nation are thus "viewed as means calculated to achieve national goals and purposes." Such actions are interpreted as solutions to domestic problems such that the "explanation of rational action consists of showing what goal the nation was pursuing in committing the action and how in the light of that goal the action was the most reasonable choice." The implication is that important policy decisions have big causes, that large organizations perform important actions to serve substantial purposes. Analysts employing this framework may disagree sharply on which causes, which reasons, and which purposes are associated with particular governmental decisions, but the similarity of their purposive analytic orientation is striking (Allison, 1968, 1ff.).

The basic unit of analysis in such work is the government's choice of strategy. The central concepts include the government as actor, governmental goals, alternative solutions, calculation, and consequences. These characteristic concepts are employed in a distinctive pattern of inference.

As Allison suggests, "if a nation or state or city has specific objectives, it will choose the optimal means towards those objectives." Conversely, if the "nation chooses an action or makes a decision, its goals can be inferred by calculating what are the ends towards which those acts constitute optimum means" (1968, 9). The result is a type of explanatory logic in which the knowledge of either goals or actions leads to an explanation of the other. Portraying governments as rational actors thus involves a characteristic model of description, explanation, and (one could show) prediction and evaluation.

Had the question of Medicare's origins been raised in organizational or bargaining terms, both the formulation and solution of the puzzle would have been different. From an organizational perspective, the question of Medicare's origins would have focused on the process by which health insurance for the aged arose as a political issue. Such an analysis would have characterized the relevant organizational units concerned with health and the aged, their standard ways of receiving, generating, and interpreting information, and their ordinary rules of decision for political strategy. Also, Chapter 1 would have dealt extensively with the organizational setting of the Medicare strategy; the central issue would have been, How is it that the shift in health insurance strategy took place? The relevant answer would have been not so much reasons why that decision made sense but rather why those reasons made sense to the organizational actors and how that led them to take this different posture toward the problems and possibilities of health insurance in American politics. Organizational analysis would emphasize that information on the aged was more readily available to organizations like the Federal Security Agency, a group charged with responsibility for the aged generally, and social security beneficiaries particularly. The reasons for concentrating on the aged would, from this view, be very different from the reasons why the aged warranted, in an objective analysis, special health concern.

My purpose here is not to treat alternative analytic frameworks as mutually exclusive. They are less discrete than that, and the analysis of a topic like Medicare's origins inevitably mixes elements of a number of analytic approaches. But I do want to emphasize the focus of attention in Chapter 1. It was on the decision to adopt a Medicare strategy and differed from the organizational analyst's interest in how a particular set of complex events takes place. Students of bureaucratic bargaining would have raised still different questions about Medicare's origins as a public issue. They would treat the Medicare strategy decision as part of an ongoing policy contest in which the most stubborn advocates of the Truman health proposals were defeated by the proponents of incrementalism. Detailed information about the actors involved and the governmental atmosphere in which the Ewing plan emerged would be required for this type of analysis. Very little appears in this book about the structure of the Federal Security Agency, its relations with the Truman staff, and its connections with congressional health insurance advocates.

It is precisely that sort of evidence that permits characterizing a bargaining game out of which a strategic choice emerges. Such a view not only stresses political victors and losers, but treats decisions as part of an ongoing struggle. The shift to a Medicare approach is but one stage in a fluid policy development; the incentives of key actors to promote or oppose this shift would be part of an overall portrait of the health-politics field. Some of this perspective was evident in the detail included in Chapter 1. The prominent position within the Federal Security Agency of such longtime social security experts as Wilbur Cohen and I. S. Falk helped to explain the availability of a social insurance alternative to the Truman plan. (It should be remembered that both these officials were advocates of general health insurance, but less sanguine than others as to its political feasibility.) The access Cohen and Falk had to Oscar Ewing constituted a crucial bargaining advantage for those seeking a limited, but more politically appealing health insurance initiative. The difference between explaining why health insurance for the aged made sense and why that decision was adopted should by now be more apparent. In Chapter 1 we permitted the answer to the former question to serve as a parsimonious proxy for the latter.

THE RESPONSES OF MEDICARE, 1952–64: THE ORGANIZATIONAL PROCESS MODEL

The second topic of this book is the fate of Medicare proposals *after* the Ewing-Truman decision. We were interested in the contestants about Medicare and the nature of the contest over time. Here our concern for describing and accounting for a *pattern* of organizational behavior makes the rational actor framework less useful. The immediate organizational problems of concerned pressure groups at this point took precedence over the social problems of the aged to which the advocates of Medicare had drawn attention. In discussing this aspect of the problem, we were less interested in Medicare as a rational response to the problems of the elderly and more concerned with the use made of their woes by pressure group antagonists. In characterizing the Medicare contest, we concentrated on the major organizational units concerned and, implicitly, employed some of the characteristic features of what has been called the organizational process model (Allison, 1968, 3).

Explanations in organizational terms typically "focus on the pattern of statements, directives, and actions of relevant agencies and departments." A central assumption is that organizations change slowly, that behavior in time $t + 1$ will resemble that of time t. Predictions thus are based on the "structure, programs, and past behavior of the relevant organizations" (Allison, 1968, 22). Throughout, our central concern is how certain patterns of activity take place in the special organizations we call government.

Chapters 2 and 3 stress that both the contest and the contestants over Medicare remained remarkably stable in the period 1952–64, "two well-defined camps with opposing views, camps with few individuals who were impartial or uncommitted" (cf. Wildavsky, 1962, 304). The breadth of the conflict over Medicare was illustrated by the large number of concerned groups (often otherwise not involved with health issues) and their ideological polarization. The disputes over Medicare had recurring, predictable features even as the specific proposals in question changed substantially. The disputants—like adversaries in open class conflict—called upon crystallized attitudes and positions and expressed them in distinctive ways to identify problems and frame remedies. The stability in Medicare demands and reactions permitted a relatively static description of group conflict on this issue.

The stereotypical and static quality of the fight over Medicare is more readily understandable when one considers the size and character of the parties to it.[1] Large national associations like the AMA and AFL-CIO have widely dispersed component parts; they function in part as Washington lobbyists for issues affecting the interests of widely disparate members. Hence, they must seek common denominators of sentiment that will satisfy the organization's leading actors without antagonizing large bodies of more passive members. Such large organizations are specialized, with full-time staffs devoted to preparing responses to public policy questions when the occasion arises and in the direction dictated by past organizational attitudes. These attitudes are slow to change and help account for the predictable way in which sides were taken on various Medicare proposals over time. Intelligence and research were weapons in a long struggle between groups that distrusted each other. Hence, it is not surprising that the debate was stable; mutually incompatible positions on health insurance arose in part from the maintenance needs of large-scale organizations (and their leaders).

An organizational perspective was appropriate for analyzing the *pattern* of Medicare debates and debaters. In dealing with that pattern it was useful to concentrate on the predictable behavior of the large pressure groups involved. Students of organizations know that such collectivities do not behave like individuals. Organizations filter information in ways persons do not. They seek means to maintain themselves over time not characteristic of individual behavior. The conjunction of the routine behavior of many individuals in organizational settings has results in public policy for which one cannot account by looking only at the activities of isolated individuals.

Other questions could have been raised about the long fight over Medicare. Had one concentrated on explaining a particular response to a particular proposal (the 1961 congressional battle, for instance), it would have been more appropriate to stress individual actions and the individual bargaining that characterized that episode. That was precisely the approach used in discussing 1961 events and, in particular, the 1965 legislative outcome.

THE 1965 LEGISLATION: THE BUREAUCRATIC POLITICS MODEL

The enactment of Medicare was treated in earlier chapters primarily as the result of a bargaining game in which none of the relevant executive, legislative, or pressure-group players could fully control the outcome. The key actors—Mills and Byrnes of the Ways and Means Committee, Cohen of HEW, Long and Anderson of the Senate Finance Committee, the AMA, and the labor leaders—all had different conceptions of the problem at hand. They had different stakes in the outcome of the legislative struggle and different terms on which they were willing to compromise.

Not only was bargaining stressed—both explicit and tacit—but also the decentralized nature of the American political process. It was never clear at what stage in the legislative process major alterations were or were not possible. The statutory result could not be interpreted solely as the product of the administration's intentions. Rather, it emerged as the outcome of a long, complicated struggle and the law in its final form was not one that any of the major actors intended at the outset.

The bureaucratic politics framework considers "domestic policy" to consist of *outcomes* of a series of overlapping "bargaining games" arranged hierarchically within the national government. Two descriptive emphases are involved: that governments are made up of disparate, decentralized organizations headed by leaders with unequal power, and that such leaders, in the course of policymaking, engage in bargaining. These players, operating with different perspectives and different priorities, struggle for preferred outcomes with the power at their disposal. Explanations in this third model proceed from descriptions of the "position and power of the principal players" and concentrate on the "understandings and misunderstandings which determine the outcome of the game" (Allison, 1968, 3).

The basic unit of analysis is the decentralized bargaining game played by relatively autonomous actors. The focal concepts include bargaining strategies, roles, moves, stakes, trade-offs, tactics, and conventions (or rules of the game). Explanations that employ this framework typically draw upon the stakes and interests the actors bring to disputes about particular policy issues. The decisions and actions of governments constitute outcomes in the "sense that what happens is not chosen as a solution to a problem" but is rather the result of "political bargaining among a number of independent players, of compromise, coalition, competition, and confusion among government officials many of whom are focusing on different faces of the issue." The actions of government—the sum of the "behavior of representatives of a government" involved in a policy issue—"is rarely intended by any individual or group." From this characterization of policymaking come distinctive patterns of inference, rules of explanation such as "where you stand depends on where you sit." Moreover, important government decisions are not viewed as the result of a single game. Rather, what the government does is a "collage of individual acts, outcomes of minor and major games, and foul-ups." The understanding of that cumulative process requires piece-by-piece disaggregation of the policymaking. What moves the process, in any event, is not simply the "reasons which support a course of action, nor the routines of organizations which enact an alternative, but the power and skill of proponents and opponents of the action in question" (Allison, 1968, 26ff.).

Treating statues as bargaining outcomes requires the sort of detailed characterization of individual styles, interests, and position that Chapter 4 presented. Actors like Mills, for instance, no longer asked in January, 1965, whether it was preferable that the U.S. government provide hospital and nursing home insurance for the aged under social security. That much was a foregone conclusion, which shaped the behavior of an adaptive committee chairman like Mills. He could in 1965 be a reluctant bystander or an adroit manager of legislation that in another setting he would have preferred to block. Mills always adjusted to legislative certainty and tried to take charge of the form that the inevitable takes. Cutting back on the administration's proposal in 1965 was an extraordinarily difficult alternative, given that the problems of the aged had been identified in a way for which the "input" of H.R. 1 was at best a partial solution. Moreover, scrimping on the aged when legislation was imminent was more difficult than preventing any Medicare action whatsoever in the period before 1965. These were the types of considerations that dominated the presentation of Chapter 4: evidence about the rules of the legislative game, the stakes involved, and the radically altered nature of the 1965 setting. The bargaining that took place should not be allowed to obscure the vital fact that the election of 1964 had given all the actors less to bargain about.

We have thus far concentrated on showing how different analytic approaches lead to distinguishable sets of questions about public policy developments like Medicare legislation. It should be added that they also make a difference in the evaluations, recommendations, and predictions one makes about public policy. Consider some of the predictive and prescriptive differences that would emerge from alternative approaches to the explanation of the Medicare statute. The analyst who viewed Medicare legislation as the national solution to a pressing social problem would expect (and predict) that periodic adjustments would be made to make the program a more efficient instrument to cope with the health and financial problems of the aged. He would expect monitoring of the program as part of the effort to increase the level of achievement of the original national goal.[2]

Contrast these predictions with those a bargaining analyst would make on the basis of Chapter 4. He would expect future outcomes to vary with what one might call the deal of the electoral cards. Since the innovations of 1965 were so much the result of the atypical partisan makeup of the 88th Congress, he would predict less innovation in more typical Congresses. He would not expect the Committee on Ways and Means, for instance, to preoccupy itself with improving the program, or to seek aggressively alternative means to meet the health needs of other Americans not assisted by Medicare.

Political recommendations would be equally different. One could imagine problem-solvers trying to convince the congressional committee that new difficulties, such as higher medical prices, have arisen for the aged, or that more serious health and financial problems are being felt by the disadvantaged and poor. The emphasis here would be on identifying the social ills for which national action is required. Students of bargaining would offer different recommendations. They would stress continued efforts to reshape the Committee on Ways and Means, taking cues from the "packing" of the committee after 1961. They would advise political investments of this kind, rather than a search for problems, as the best means of insuring action on health problems we are already well aware of. Viewed from the anti-Medicare perspective, bargaining students would firmly recommend prevention of these long-term investments. These illustrations—admittedly brief and elliptical—are examples of the differences that analytic lenses may make in what we see, predict, and recommend about public policy.

PROCESSES AND POLICY IN AMERICAN POLITICS: THE CASE OF MEDICARE

The preceding analytic discussion raised issues about studying American public policy that were not explicitly discussed in the case study itself. In turning to the relation between Medicare politics and more general characterizations of American political life, I will try to make systematic the observations and connections that were intermittently raised in the first five chapters. There is a substantial literature on American political processes and considerable evidence of what is taken to be distinctive about the politics of some subject matter (tariffs or housing) or some broad class of policies (regulatory or distributive). The first part of the following discussion will compare Medicare findings with these broader generalizations; its aim is to present evidence why some generalizations appear plausible, though, by its nature, case study material cannot constitute a definitive test. The second part will compare the substance of Medicare policy with other views of the typical allocative and redistributive policies generated in American politics.

Political scientists have expended great efforts in recent years trying to specify the ways by which different issues are raised, disputed, coped with, and sometimes "solved." Lowi (1964) has provided a typology for discriminating among public policies that usefully categorizes the Medicare case. He describes three major patterns of political conflict that are said to be associated with three different types of public policies—*distributive, regulative,* and *redistributive.* Distributive policies, which parcel out public benefits to interested parties, provoke a stable alliance of diverse groups that seek portions of the pork barrel. Regulative policies, which constrain the relations among competing groups and persons, provide incentives for shifting coalitions, pluralistic competition, and the standard forms of compromise. Redistributive policies, which reallocate benefits and burdens among broad socioeconomic population groups, foster polarized and enduring conflict in which large national pressure groups play central roles.

Lowi characterizes three patterns of conflict, but identifies them by their putative cause—the type of policy.[3] It is clear that actual policies are never so distinct. All public programs redistribute resources, but most are not primarily attempts to do so. Likewise, all government programs depend upon an ultimate capacity to regulate the conduct of citizens, but most do not make such regulation their prime object. And almost all government programs involve the distribution of goods and services among different groups, though the question of which county or which social class should receive them is not always salient. But whatever the cause of the pattern of conflict, one can assess which pattern is illustrated by individual policy conflicts like Medicare.

The conflict over Medicare mirrors the political processes Lowi identifies with redistributive policies. The themes of that conflict—the threat of "big government," the interests of the have-nots vs. the haves—illustrate the cluster of issues that arise when a policy question "involves the issue of whether broad categories of persons are to be better or worse off" (Lowi, 1964, 689). The debate over Medicare was in fact cast in the terms of class conflict, of socialized medicine vs. the voluntary "American way," of private enterprise and local control against "the octopus of the federal government." Moreover, though the program most immediately affected the aged, physicians, and hospitals, broad strata of the population were directly or indirectly involved—the families of the aged, all present social security contributors, and the entire health industry.

Not only the themes of the conflict, but the antagonists and their adversary methods illustrate what might be called "class conflict" politics. The dispute over Medicare reenacted the polarization that characterized earlier fights over national health insurance. The leading adversaries—national business, health, and labor organizations—participated in open communication (though not to their mutual enlightenment) and brought into the opposing camps a large number of groups whose interests were not directly affected by the Medicare outcome. In the process, ideological charges and countercharges dominated public discussion, and each side seemed to regard compromise as unacceptable. In the end, the electoral changes of 1964 reallocated power in such a way that the opponents were overruled. Compromise was involved in the detailed features of the Medicare program, but the enactment itself did not constitute a compromise outcome for the adversaries. In all these respects, Medicare politics differed from the discrete and localized pursuit of pork barrel benefits or the shifting coalitions and compromises of regulatory politics.

Battles like Medicare are fought in public but settled in private. The national pressure groups concerned made enormous and costly efforts to define the dispute over Medicare in ways acceptable to their members. But within the government bureaucracy, there were continuing efforts to articulate and balance these rival claims in the legislation proposed to the Congress. The consultation was sometimes explicit and detailed, as when the AFL-CIO and the Blue Cross Association met regularly with HEW officials during the early 1960s. In other cases, consideration of group interest was tacit and intermittent, particularly in the case of the AMA. Overall, the executive proposals sent to Congress reflected a typical pattern: major compromises were built into Medicare bills proposed by the executive branch, anticipating the pressure group claims that would otherwise have to be balanced in the Congress.

The role of Congress in dealing with policy problems like Medicare is to "ratify the agreement" that arises out of "the bureaucracy and the class agents represented there" (Lowi, 1964, 171). Had Medicare passed in 1964, this characterization of executive preeminence would have been fully warranted; the bill of that year was a hesitantly redistributive version of hospital insurance for the aged, designed to assist the aged but shaped to serve and meet the economic demands of insurance companies and the hospitals as well. The fact that Congress unexpectedly added physician insurance to the program enacted in 1965 represents a departure from the modal processes of redistributive politics, a departure that can be explained by the extraordinary electoral context of 1965. The significant changes in the administration bill were made almost exclusively in committee deliberations. Minor adjustments arose from Senate debate, none from the House, where the vote on Medicare took place without amendment. The executive branch was throughout the locus of legislative planning and drafting; the peculiarities of the 1965 Congress should not obscure the patterns of the preceding decade.

The polarization elicited by issues like Medicare shapes the behavior of all the interested pressure groups. Medicare was one of those issues that separates the "money-providing" and "service-demanding" groups in a society—a division that "cuts closer than any other along class lines" (Lowi, 1964, 707, 711). This promotes cohesion among groups that otherwise have much to disagree about; the existence of a common fear promotes a public united front. So, for instance, the conflicting interests of the American Hospital Association (certain to be assisted by Medicare's underwriting of the hospital expenses of the aged) and the American Medical Association (violently opposed to Medicare, despite its members' short-run economic interests) were muted through most of the fight over Medicare. Hospital Association officials felt constrained to take the "health industry's" position against Medicare, though in private (and in meetings with HEW), their willingness to go along with the legislation was apparent. The health industry's public opposition was fused with that of almost every national commercial, industrial, and right-wing group in American politics. The united front of "service-demanders" was equally apparent in the Medicare fight. The ultimate consumers—the aged and their organizations—were sometimes overshadowed in the procession of "liberal" professional, labor, and service organizations championing their cause.

Finally, the processes of Medicare politics involved stabilizing and centralizing conflict in ways characteristic of redistributive disputes (Lowi, 1964, 715). The initiation of Medicare demands in the early 1950s—when the issue was simply whether the social security system would provide 60 days of hospital insurance for its beneficiaries—revealed the pattern of conflict that would follow. Specters of the future—fearful or hopeful—dominated the ideological charges of the national pressure groups. The liberal-conservative split that emerged remained stable throughout, with few defectors as the proposals shifted. The Department of Health, Education and Welfare centralized much of the battle. Congress, whose fiscal committees are short of staff and unequipped to conduct independent research on health affairs, "listened" to the repetitive debates and, in the end, ratified the administration's bill, adding its own special imprint.

Most Medicare bills did not propose massive redistribution of income, and in this sense the association of Medicare with Lowi's redistributive politics may appear problematic. But the central feature of the Medicare dispute was whether the federal government should engage in whatever limited redistribution Medicare proposals entailed. The fight centered on whether the redistribution was warranted (were the aged needy enough?), the instrument of change (charity or insurance?), and the sources of financing (general revenues or social security taxes?). This redistributive frame of reference determined the shape of the conflict, not the scale of redistribution that would in fact be involved.

Medicare thus appears to be an instance of a much larger class of conflicts in American politics associated with issues of income redistribution and zero-sum political conflicts. Our findings about Medicare can be used, however, to illustrate more than classificatory generalizations. More general questions—involving the structure of power in the United States—are relevant. What was the role of public opinion in this major public policy choice? How influential were pressure groups and whom did they seek to pressure?

The Medicare case illustrates the comparative irrelevance of mass public opinion in federal policymaking (Key, 1961; Bauer, de Sola Pool, & Dexter, 1963). Public support for health insurance under social security declined slightly as remedial proposals were more specifically defined. Polls revealed less support as the probabilities of legislative action increased, a finding comparable to Meranto's (1967) in the case of federal aid to education and consistent with more general conclusions about the nature of mass opinion. When pollsters shift from asking general questions about the need for social action to specific questions about particular remedies, support seems to fragment. In any event, the architects of Medicare never sought public views on legislative details, but rather were after (in V. O. Key's memorable term) a "permissive consensus" (1961). They sought and discovered overwhelming majorities of respondents ready to acknowledge the comparatively severe health and financial problems of the aged. They found substantial majorities willing to support a "solution" to these difficulties through the social security system. In short, they found their "problem" to be credible and their remedial instrument "legitimate." But as one would expect, the polls revealed substantial ignorance of the details of the standard Medicare proposals, and an important and mistaken tendency to assume that Medicare referred to comprehensive medical and hospital insurance (see Chapter 4).

The discrepancy between public understanding and the actual Medicare proposal highlights the limited role of mass opinion in this policy area. Public support for "doing something" about the health problems of the aged declined as the question became more specific, from nearly 70 percent support for federal action in general to about 55 percent support for specific Kennedy and Johnson bills. But support, at either level of specificity, did not substantially vary with the prospects of congressional action. No change in public attitude accompanied the enactment of the Kerr-Mills program in 1960. Likewise in 1965 there was no noticeable change in public attitude once electoral changes ensured some sort of Medicare legislation.

It might be argued that massive public sympathy with the problems of the aged and mass approval of the social security system were the necessary but not sufficient conditions for the enactment of Medicare. Specifying the impact of such opinion on the policymaking process is, nonetheless, extremely difficult. Those who assume government leaders are limited by what they think the public will buy are perhaps confusing an effort to avoid conflict with groups like the AMA with an attempt to "get around" alleged public preferences. (See the exclusion of surgical benefits from the Medicare proposals from 1958 on, Chapter 3.) In the end, public opinion of Medicare's benefits played an indirect and unanticipated role in the expansion of the program. Misunderstandings about the meaning of Medicare—the impression that both physician's and hospital bills would be covered—provided advocates of broader benefits with unexpected political resources. But the way in which this informational discrepancy was taken into account was haphazard, a process of social choice in which critics of Medicare's misleading publicity were used for purposes quite unlike those they accepted.

The long, expensive, and extensive efforts of pressure groups to affect the Medicare outcome should not lead us to confuse the volume or intensity of their publicity with influence. The failure to distinguish group participation from group influence has in fact been a conceptual weakness of the pluralist model of pressure group politics. Lowi points out that the "proof" of a pluralistic American political structure is all too often entailed by the definitional and conceptual assumptions of the analyst:

Issues are chosen for research because conflict made them public; group influence is found because groups so often share in definition of the issue and have taken positions that are more or less congruent with the out-comes. An indulged group was influential, and a deprived group was uninfluential; but that leaves no room for group irrelevance. (1964, 681)

This conclusion is abundantly illustrated in the attribution of influ-ence to the American Medical Association. Medicare defeats during the 1962–64 period were typically viewed as AMA victories, even though AMA actions were not the chief reason for legislative inaction. To be sure, the AMA did enjoy influence in shaping the Medicare debate. The pattern of Medicare proposals over time illustrated the capacity of the AMA to influence the agenda of discussion and to limit the alternatives policymakers would suggest. Perhaps the most vivid illustration of this preemptive power was the deliberate exclusion of physician insurance from Medicare proposals after 1958. However, if the limits of debate were in part a result of AMA influence, legislative decisions were not. The succession of Medicare defeats arose from congressional power dis-tributions whose effects the AMA could enjoy but whose character the AMA could only marginally affect. The effort to build a coalition in the pre-1965 period took into account AMA objections, but the decisive elec-toral shift of 1965 illuminated the true basis of past Medicare defeats. The congressional structure—inordinately responsive to southern De-mocratic inclinations—was substantially changed for the moment, and Medicare legislation quickly followed. Just as one should distinguish the causes of the enactment of a Medicare bill from the reasons for par-ticular provisions, so one should distinguish the capacity to shape dis-cussion from the ability to produce legislative outcomes.

Much of the alleged power of pressure groups, as shown by recent political science literature, is the product of the imagination and imagery of contending groups. The 1961 battle over Medicare vividly illustrates this process. The Democratic administration helped create an image of a powerful AMA to call attention away from its own inca-pacity to make Congress (and especially the Ways and Means Commit-tee) do its bidding. Much pressure group effort, in any case, is spent in bolstering group supporters, not changing congressional minds. Such efforts, with the possible exception of regulatory politics, typically involves "inter- reaction with people on the same side" of an issue (Bauer et al., 1963, 398). This was unquestionably the case during the long Medicare conflict, where the two leading group antagonists—the AFL-CIO and the AMA—never had the occasion or inclination for prelegislative bargaining. The executive bureaucracy played a broker's role between these "opposing sides," tacitly incorporating compromises into legislative proposals, particularly in the final stages of enactment. HEW officials like Cohen and Ball consulted labor organizations and the health professions in ways public debate did not allow. The opponents investigated on its merits very little of what each other claimed; there was an overwhelming tendency to bifurcate the universe into friends and enemies and to "learn" only from friends. Pressure groups used the imagined (or real) power of their opponents to rally support for their "side." The massive propaganda efforts of both the AMA and AFL-CIO were never judged by their actual effects on crucial political leaders. Rather, each side indicated the need for solidarity and the seriousness of the conflict by publicizing the propaganda expenditures of its adversary.

It must not be assumed that redistributive social welfare issues alone generate the kind of polarized ideological conflict we have been describing. Redistributive issues may well make up the bulk of such conflicts, but they do not comprise the class. There is a strikingly close parallel between the political processes evidenced in Medicare and those, for example, in public power conflicts in America. Wildavsky (1962) has characterized the latter conflict in much the same way as in the Lowi typology and illustrated by Medicare. The obvious difference between disputes over public power (the public role in electricity, gas, etc.) and federal health insurance should not obscure either the similar style of conflict or their common ideological roots. Both issues involve the legitimacy of federal action and, by implication, limits on private initiative. In this respect, they differ from pork barrel disputes over how much one area or group or another receives in public expenditures and services. They differ as well from regulatory issues in which, once legislation is effective, the conflicts focus on the burdens and benefits of particular governmental rules. The most bitter fight over Medicare and such public power issues as Dixon-Yates is at the level of principle, not particular burdens and benefits. The question whether the government should be acting at all is central, and in turn calls forth the ideological polarization and national pressure group activity previously discussed. Consider Wildavsky's generalizations about Dixon-Yates (1962, 304–5) alongside the political processes that characterized Medicare:

1. A very large percentage of the active participants in the controversy divided into well-defined camps with opposing views (the AMA-led opposition versus the AFL-CIO–led proponents). Active individuals who were impartial or uncommitted or who dissented from the two major views were rare.

2. Professional bureaucracies developed with full-time staffs who made a career out of fighting on the issue and there were public figures who made their reputations in this field (e.g., Wilbur Cohen, with long-term social security experts like Ball and Wolkstein, joined by Nelson

Cruikshank of the AFL-CIO and William Hutton of the Senior Citizen Organization on one side; and on the other, Dr. Edward Annis of the AMA, and many others, supported by the substantial staffs of the NAM, Chamber of Commerce, American Farm Bureau Federation, etc.).

3. Since the opposing groups had long since been formed, their active members were acutely aware of who was on their side and who was on the opposing team (e.g., the immediate HEW impulse to reject the Byrnes plan in early 1965, Chapter 4).

4. Personal contacts were largely restricted to individuals on the same side (the case throughout in Medicare, except for some of the HEW leaders).

5. Having good reason to believe that they had "heard it all before," the disputants were disinclined to listen to arguments on the other side (e.g., participants talking past one another in public hearings throughout the period 1958–65).

6. Opponents had in reserve prepared responses ready to be activated whenever the occasion demanded (e.g., the responses of Medicare proponents to the notion of need, and the familiar arguments against the alleged vices of the social security system).

7. Views on this issue were frequently held with considerable passion, leading to a strong tendency to oversimplify, to regard events and personalities in terms of black and white. One's opponents were regarded as inherently suspect of all kinds of devious actions, while one's supporters were considered to be above suspicion (e.g., the familiar characterization of Cohen as a "Czar" by his critics, and the HEW suspicions of AMA initiatives in 1965).

8. Involvement in the controversy was sufficiently intense for the participants to use a large part of their resources to secure a favorable outcome (e.g., lobbying expenditures, and the proportion of time spent in 1965 on Medicare matters by the top ten HEW officials).

9. While the participants may have had a direct economic stake in the controversy, they came in time to feel that more was involved than money and property. The conflict then took on an ideological hue, with victory or defeat seen in terms of overriding general principles that must not be sacrificed (e.g., the broad appeals on both sides of Medicare to norms of federalism, the "American way," tax policy, the dignity of the aged, the "welfare state," collectivism, etc.).

The issues that generate such broad ideological polarization range beyond health insurance and public ownership of power plants. Studies of the legislative dispute over federal aid to education have recently documented similar features (Munger and Fenno, 1962; Meranto, 1967;

Eidenberg and Morey, 1969). Past disputes over public housing have activated similar antagonists and methods of antagonizing (Friedman, 1968). But not all, or even most, political conflicts assume this form; generally it is when the legislative issue is the broad redistribution of power and income (money, services, and authority) that the quest for initiative or for veto coalitions generates the processes of polarization. The site and agents of such conflict clearly vary from issue to issue. Sometimes the dispute is lodged in the executive (Dixon-Yates) and extensively covered by the media. In other cases, conflict and concessions are brought out in congressional committees, with the executive branch playing a somewhat more passive role (public housing and some welfare legislation). Within Congress, issues vary as to whether amendment and substantial adjustments take place through floor action (education legislation and appropriations, for example) or in committee. The important point is not the site of such conflicts, but the parties that fight them out and the issues that generate them. What constitutes the limits of this class of political conflicts is an important empirical question that individual case studies cannot answer. One may not assume from the evidence given here that redistributive issues are always class-based and ideological, or that ideological polarization always arises about the likely redistributive impact of a given policy. But one can conclude that explicitly redistributive issues strikingly generate the sort of conflict that characterized Medicare politics.

Neither Wildavsky nor Lowi, however, tell us anything about the typical outcome of such conflicts. The analysis of the content of ideologically divisive policies does not logically follow from generalizations about processes of conflict. An independent inquiry is required concerning the kinds of policy outcomes one might expect from the disputes Wildavsky and Lowi have described.

MEDICARE AND THE CHARACTER OF AMERICAN SOCIAL POLICY

This section will briefly compare Medicare's programmatic structure with other American public policies, particularly other social welfare programs. This concern with the content of public policy responds to an impulse that other American political scientists have noted and encouraged. Ranney rightly contends that "at least since 1945 most American political scientists have focused their professional attention mainly on the *processes* by which public policies are made and have shown relatively little concern with their *contents*" (1968, 3). Ranney is at pains to distinguish programmatic intentions and practices from the consequences they produce, to separate a policy and its outcome. The relation between policies (their intended objects, goals, programmatic practices) and political outcomes (affected persons, principles served, and subsequent practices) is an empirical issue of great interest. The study in this book has taken Medicare policy (in the above sense) as its subject and cannot hope to comment extensively on the consequences that followed its adoption and implementation. Nonetheless, my present purpose is to consider the policy contents of Medicare not for what they tell us about American political processes but to compare the nature of that policy itself with others.

There is no need to repeat my previous descriptions of the Medicare program: its noncomprehensive health insurance benefits, regressive financing, aged beneficiaries, centralized and nondiscretionary administration, and non-means-tested eligibility features. Rather, two central issues warrant comment here. The first is the appropriateness of the classificatory criteria that permitted such a description; the second is the generality of this type of programmatic result.

Policies may be described by their beneficiaries (the poor, farmers, widows, etc.), their financing (regressive, proportional, progressive), their administrative structure (centralized or decentralized, discretionary, or nondiscretionary), their source of entitlement (earned or unearned), the extent of their departure from past practices (radical or incremental). Little is gained from debate over which descriptive set is most useful; that depends upon the purpose of the inquirer. But much is gained—for those interested in the burdens and benefits of American public policy—by characterizing who is to benefit from and who is to administer a given policy. These questions can be applied to any policy at any level of government. They thus permit generalizations about programs that are quite different in the goods or services they distribute.

Friedman (1969) has used such a scheme (see Table 5.1) in characterizing American housing policy in the recent past. He identifies two social welfare policy types as "middle-class" and "charity" programs. Such emotive terms are not necessary to observe that Medicare represents the former type and that the Medicare debate centered on the choice between these two models.

Not all social policies represent one or the other of these polar types, but some, such as the social insurance provisions of the Social Security Act of 1935 and Medicare, are pure middle-class programs. In such programs, "benefits tend to be a matter of right; eligibilities are earned; benefits are restitutionary; the means-test is avoided" (Friedman, 1969, 247). The characteristics of "charity laws" like Medicaid or Kerr-Mills "are flatly reversed." A review of the contrast between the Forand and

Table 5.1.   American Housing Policy Classified by Beneficiary

Criteria	*Middle-Class Program*	*Charity Program*
Beneficiaries	Broad demographic unit, not selected by test of means	"Needy" persons selected by test of means
Benefits	Earned, noncomprehensive for given problem	Given, not earned, and more comprehensive
Financing	Regressive, as with earmarked Social Security taxes	General revenues, more progressive source
Administration	Centralized, nondiscretionary and clerklike, with highly developed rules of entitlement	Discretionary, decentralized

Kerr-Mills proposals would support the interpretation that these two conceptions of appropriate social policy were at stake.

The extent to which other social policies fall into this dichotomous pattern can only be answered through investigation. Exceptions come immediately to mind. The old-age assistance program in California, for instance, is widely known for the dignified way in which beneficiaries are selected and for the clerklike character of program administration. The income-tested veterans pension is, likewise, a means-tested program that has little of the degrading and discretionary character commonly associated with public assistance, and is an example of centralized federal programs for "needy" persons. But the issue is not whether exceptions exist, but what constitute the general patterns of social policy. This case study attests only to the plausibility of the Friedman classification.

Friedman is interested as well in the determinants of each type of social welfare legislation. Public assistance—particularly general relief at the local level and federal-state assistance to families with dependent children (AFDC)—typify what have been termed "charity" programs. That is not meant to suggest that such programs are charitably run, but that means-tested programs are associated with local discretion and general tax funds. Friedman suggests that the effort to elicit wide support for programs that avoid the connotations of "welfare" almost inevitably, in American politics, produce middle-class legislative models. The designated clientele (needy persons rather than a demographic unit) is the causal key. Programs for both the rich and the poor make means tests less relevant, and local administration less crucial. Restitutionary programs are legitimated by past acts, not present income; they avoid the moral choices between deserving and undeserving recipients by designating recipients in terms of past contributions or neutral demographic attributes. Finally, the clientele theory assumes that the particular type of benefit (cash or kind) does not determine the form of the policy, or its likely character over time. There are, Friedman would argue, two major types of "social welfare policy," not distinctive health, housing, education, and cash-transfer policies.

The foregoing remarks apply primarily to types of social welfare laws, not patterns of policy consequences. Not only may implementation deviate from statutory intention, but statutes and programs may distribute different types of benefits. Edelman (1964) has rightly distinguished between the symbolic burdens and benefits that statutes may provide and the tangible assistance (and deprivation) that operating programs in fact distribute. Not all statutes are strictly enforced, and "preambles to legislation" can be used to "symbolize concern and hoodwink people with symbolic reassurance that all will be well once the law is on the books" (Mitchell and Mitchell, 1969, 162). The passage of Medicare unquestionably involved such symbolic reassurance. But its implementation distributed intended financial benefits to the aged even though all might not be well once the law was on the books. In addition, however, there were substantial unintended beneficiaries from the programmatic practices of the Social Security Administration and the health insurance industry.

The most striking development was the extent to which Medicare benefited those who opposed it most. Medicare was advocated as an insurance measure, not as an instrument of reform in the organization and delivery of personal health services. Though physician services were typically excluded from Medicare proposals, the AMA was Medicare's most hostile critic and the most serious symbolic loser from its enactment. But physicians have received substantial income supplements from the Medicare program thus far, as have critics in the nursing home and hospital industries. The cooperation of health businesses was required, and Medicare was clearly intended to assist hospitals (through the improved capacity of their aged patients to pay) and insurance companies (relieved of the financially onerous task of insuring the aged at low premiums). But the scale of such assistance (and its extension to physicians) was unappreciated by most of those who participated in the legislative process. Those who think health groups wrung such concessions as a price of legislative cooperation confuse intended with unintended consequences, and explicit with tacit bargaining. Most of the generous features of Medicare were attempts to forestall difficulties, not respond to them. And the price of such generosity, four years later, prompted the Department of Health, Education and Welfare to warn about the "extreme urgency of the [health cost] situation, [and] to encourage steps to arrest the inflation that is paralyzing us." Such price inflation was not intended, even by those in the Johnson administration, who most understood that the bitter Medicare bill must be sweetened for its opponents in the health industry.

Since the enactment of Medicare, the prices of hospital and physician services have risen markedly. The arrangements for paying physicians were more generous than their lobbyists might have expected even had they participated in negotiations on methods of payment (Marmor, 1968). Physician fees have risen between 5 and 8 percent per year since the start of the program; physician incomes, nearly 11 percent per year (Somers, 1968). These increases have made American physicians among Medicare's most prominent beneficiaries. This result was not only unintended by Medicare proponents, but largely unanticipated in the course of the legislative struggle over the 1965 bill. This development suggests caution in describing public policies primarily by the benefits and beneficiaries specified in law.

The implementation of Medicare illustrates another important distinction between legislative action and policy content. When issues are moral and symbolic, as in legislative struggles over the redistribution of important resources, a great variety of attentive publics are aroused. In Medicare there were active national pressure groups representing large numbers of Americans directly or indirectly involved in the health and financial circumstances of the aged. When questions arose about Medicare's administration, some attentive groups become financially interested parties, the producer groups, involved in the production and delivery of health services. The aged remained active, of course, and along with the representatives of the AFL-CIO, have sat on advisory bodies set up by the Social Security Administration at congressional behest. The hospital, nursing home, laboratory, and physician representatives nonetheless predominate. This administrative confrontation is a relatively new experience for Medicare's Social Security Administration. SSA has "never had to deal," said one official rather sadly, "with hostile pressure groups at the administrative level." The nature of conflict changes when the political question turns to who receives tangible benefits. The Social Security system—distributing cash directly, for the most part—has never had to rely on the cooperation of hostile industries in anything but tax collection. It is in administrative politics that well-organized producers are at an advantage; their interest in symbolic issues carries over to practical struggles in ways one does not predict of general reform groups and consumer organizations. The Social Security Administration was thus unprepared to deal with economic pressure groups, especially those which, though ideologically opposed to social insurance, were nonetheless desperately interested in the benefits actually distributed by a program whose initiation they in other contexts strongly opposed.

NOTES

1. It might be objected that stereotypes and simplified images of opponents are characteristic of most political disputes. But anyone who has, for example, surveyed the hearings of regulatory bodies will recognize an attention to evidential canons never present when Medicare antagonists aired their views, whether in the press or during congressional hearings. Part of the reason, of course, is that Medicare actors were directing their remarks to a much wider audience and naturally relied on compelling symbols where complex factual presentations would have been confusing or boring.

2. This follows from the assumption that the problem was financial inability of the aged to manage their health costs. If the "problem" had been defined as coping with the demand by unions, the aged, and others for "some" health care assistance, the legislation of 1965 might well be considered a rational (and nearly complete) solution.

3. This formulation of the Lowi scheme owes much to an unpublished paper by Paul Peterson of the University of Chicago: "The Politics of Welfare," 1969.

6

Legislation to Operation
The 1965–66 Transition

The Medicare program began July 1, 1966. In the year between enactment and the eligibility for benefits, the Social Security Administration itself engaged in massive preparatory tasks. The most important of these was to contact the aged and inform them of their rights to coverage and the scope of their benefits under the program. Enrollment of the aged in the voluntary medical insurance program posed the greatest publicity problem. Aged citizens were required to sign up and begin payment of the $3 monthly premiums in order to participate. The success of this Supplementary Medical Insurance Program (formally Part B of Title 18 of the Social Security Act) obviously depended on voluntary enrollment. Accordingly, the Social Security Administration launched an intensive promotional campaign in local and national news media, directly aimed at encouraging the aged to participate. More than half of the 50 states took the initiative in enrolling and assuming the premium payments for those amongst the aged who were on the state public assistance rolls, responding understandably to the powerful financial incentives to do so. At the end of the first year of Medicare's operation, the success of the recruitment program was evident:

- Of the approximately 19 million aged citizens, 93 percent, or 17.7 million, were enrolled in the voluntary medical insurance program (Part B of Title 18).
- One in five of America's elderly had entered a hospital under the new law, and 12 million had used Part B services.
- Hospital expenses accounted for $2.5 billion of the $3.2 billion expended by the SSA for Medicare.

- On the average, patients were reimbursed for 80 percent of their hospital expenses, and Medicare covered $600 of the $750 average bill (HEW, 1967b).

In addition to enrolling potential patients, the Social Security Administration had the task of evaluating healthcare facilities whose bills they would be paying, i.e., hospitals, nursing homes, and home health agencies. The Medicare law required that medical institutions apply to participate and meet several conditions specified in the law before they could receive reimbursement for services provided to Medicare patients. Besides satisfying several standards designed to ensure a higher quality of care, the institution had to offer proof that its services were rendered on a nondiscriminatory basis, in compliance with the Civil Rights Act of 1964. These requirements frequently posed difficulties for Medicare's administrators. In many cases, those hospitals unable or unwilling to meet the certification standards were also the only facilities available to Medicare patients in their localities. On the eve of Medicare's initiation in June 1966, the nondiscriminatory requirement was embroiling the government in a well-publicized confrontation with some southern hospitals that were willing to risk exclusion from the Medicare program before desegregating their facilities. Civil rights lawyers saw Medicare as a powerful instrument for change. But the price of change was the willingness to deny (in extreme cases of noncompliance) Medicare benefits to aged persons who happened to live in areas of segregation. This dilemma was by no means resolved. Indeed, it was certain that there were hospitals in the South receiving program payments benefits whose facilities were still substantially segregated during Medicare's initial operations (Schecter, 1968).

The first year of operation brought a mixture of problems and fulfillment. The worst fears that Medicare patients would crowd the hospitals beyond their capacity were nowhere realized. Some physicians refused to cooperate, but the AMA president, Dr. James Appel, was successful in directing his organization's energies away from threats of boycotts to consultations about the terms of medical service. At the same time, the administration was pleased with the high utilization rates under the program.

The problems in administering Medicare arose not so much in connection with earlier fears as with issues that had not been widely raised at the time of passage. Some of the administrative problems were typical of large new governmental programs and hence predictable. There were delays in paying providers of service, particularly during the first summer of operations. The fact that such delay was not surprising hardly allayed the irritation of the hospitals, nursing homes, and doctors affected.

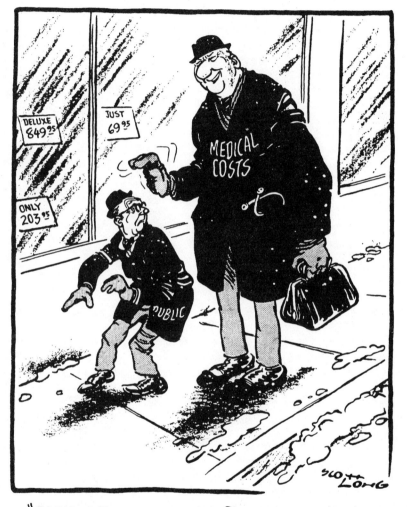

"SICK OF INFLATION? BUSTER, YOU DON'T DARE GET SICK!"

The most serious and persistent of the problems concerned the methods and costs of paying doctors and hospitals under Medicare. The statute had purposely avoided setting a specific limit on the amount a doctor could charge a Medicare patient, and specified instead that physicians were to be paid "reasonable charges." The lawmakers assumed that such charges would be higher than those customarily charged low-income patients, lest Medicare patients be treated as charity cases. The "reasonable charge" was defined as one that was "customary" for individual physicians, and no higher than the charges "prevailing" locally or those regularly paid by Medicare's payment administrators. (These fiscal intermediaries, largely but not exclusively Blue Cross for hospital expenses and Blue Shield for Part B benefits, were the decentralized agents of Medicare, another surprise of the legislative politics of enactment.) For all its seeming clarity, this standard of reasonableness was unworkable in the context of Medicare's first year. No one knew what doctors were customarily charging. There was no agreement among doctors or government officials about what constituted the upper limit of "prevailing charges." And, although Blue Shield and commercial insurance companies had evidence about their own past payments, there was no agreement about what constituted "comparable services" in "comparable circumstances."

Medicare thus began with an open-ended payment method for physicians. Doctors were as uncertain as everyone else about how the law would be construed, and fears that the insurance intermediaries would codify and freeze their definitions of "reasonable charges" gave physicians every incentive to raise their fees (Marmor, 1968). In the year between enactment of the Medicare law and its initial operation, the rate of increase in physician fees more than doubled (see Table 6.1). Some portion of that increase was undoubtedly prompted by Medicare's payment method itself, and the subsequent inflation in physician fees continued to cause serious political problems.

Hospital price increases presented the most intractable political problem for the Johnson administration. In the first year of Medicare's operation, the average daily service charge in America's hospitals increased by an unprecedented 21.9 percent (Figure 6.1). Each month the Labor Department's consumer price survey reported further

Table 6.1. Increase (%) in Physicians' Fees

	1964	1965	1966	1967
Physician fee index	2.4	3.8	7.8	6.1
Consumer price index	1.3	2.0	3.3	3.1

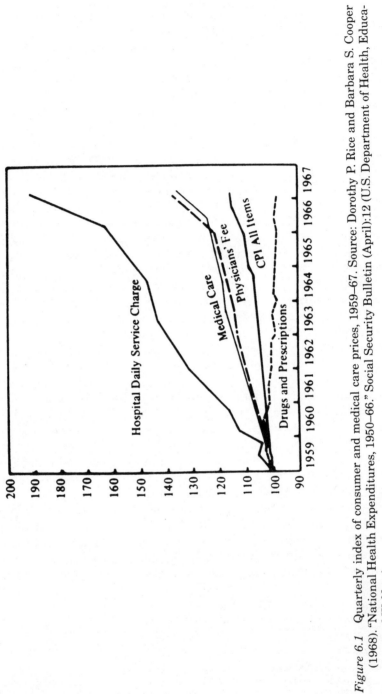

Figure 6.1 Quarterly index of consumer and medical care prices, 1959–67. Source: Dorothy P. Rice and Barbara S. Cooper (1968). "National Health Expenditures, 1950–66." Social Security Bulletin (April):12 (U.S. Department of Health, Education, and Welfare).

increases, and by the summer of 1967 President Johnson asked HEW secretary John Gardner to "study the reasons behind the rapid rise in the price of medical care and to offer recommendations for moderating that rise." Five months later Gardner reported that the Medicare program, by requiring hospitals to reexamine their costs and charges, had probably prompted many hospitals "to increase their charges" (HEW, 1967c, 2). The HEW report concluded that the question for the future "is not whether medical prices will rise, but how fast they will rise." This problem, accentuated but not caused alone by the Medicare program, would remain a worrisome political issue. In the State of the Union Address, January 17, 1968, President Johnson illustrated how the government's expanded role in financing personal health services had enlarged its responsibility for controlling price increases. Measures would be proposed, the president promised, to "stem the rising costs of medical care." While hospital costs continued to rise faster than other components of the medical care price index, the rate of increase decelerated sharply in the second year of the Medicare program from 21.9 percent in the June 1966–June 1967 period to 12.2 percent in the following year (Rice and Horowitz, 1968).

The disputes over the causes and consequences of medical inflation revealed in a striking way the differences between the politics of legislation and those of administration. Once Medicare was enacted, its publicity value dropped sharply. The press no longer had the drama of committee clashes or heated congressional debates to report to their audiences. The broad alignment of opposing economic interests that had marked the earlier Medicare debate fell apart as the issue turned from whether the government would insure the aged against health expenses to how it would do so. Groups in the medical care industry remained active, but their activities were mostly consultative and relatively unpublicized, not those of diehard ideological adversaries. Lobbyists representing hospitals, physicians, nurses, and nursing homes continually pressed their claims on the Social Security Administration and through their trade journals kept members aware of the actual workings of the Medicare program. In the process, the voice of the beneficiary (insurance consumer, patient) became less distinct. The claims of the aged insuree were less salient symbolically than those of elderly persons and their advocates pressing for the statutory redistribution of medical care. Congressmen passed on the complaints of their aged constituents, and in the case of hardships caused by the program's regulations for reimbursing physicians who directly billed their patients, there was ameliorative legislative action in 1967. Although a bill to include the disabled under Medicare provisions was defeated in 1967, no one in the Johnson administration quickly pressed for massive extensions of the program. (Within a year, however, the unabated rise in medical care prices seemed to stimulate revived interest in universal health insurance. In 1968, a labor-supported Committee for National Health Insurance was organized, and in summer of 1969 the American Hospital Association announced that it was studying the feasibility of a national health insurance plan in the United States.)

One of the fascinating features of the Medicare legislative story was the succession of new issues, unexpected outcomes, and surprising conjunctions of events. In the decades of debate over government health insurance, for example, very little attention was given to the issue of racially segregated medical services. Yet in the first weeks of the program, the question of certifying southern hospitals under Medicare took up more of the time of HEW's three top health officials than any other feature of the Medicare program. The methods of paying physicians and hospitals were among the most intractable issues that initially faced Medicare's administrators. Yet for years no one had imagined paying physicians under a Medicare program and no office of the government had thought out how this burden could best be borne. The Medicaid program of 1965—itself an unexpected congressional addition to the administration's proposal—brought with it serious controversy over exactly who would be designated as medically indigent. In California and New York, the Medicaid program faced enormous financial pressures in the first year, as the price increases and unexpectedly high utilization strained administrative budgets and prompted charges that doctors and hospitals were taking unfair advantage of the new program (Stevens and Stevens, 1974).

The disjunction between the legislative and administrative politics was not, however, surprising. The fragmentation of authority in American politics, the myriad opportunities for delaying legislative change— both entail that promoters of controversial legislation seek broad agreement among a wide variety of publics on minimal change. The consequence of this is that reformist attention became focused on creating appealing symbols and combating critical slogans: the desperation of the aged, the inadequacy of private insurance coverage, the fear of "creeping socialism." However crucial these disputes were for the legislative process, they provided no answers (indeed little discussion) about how to administer a program whose enactment was once divisive. And, with the usual American uncertainty about the timing of social legislation, it is not until programs are on the statute books that the problems of managing large-scale government innovations are directly confronted. A treatment of those problems, the resolution of which is often vital to the effectiveness of the program, is the subject of this edition's Part II.

II

THE POLITICS OF MEDICARE: 1966–99

We turn now from an account of Medicare's birth to an account of its development. As the preface noted, Part II raises a new set of questions. Medicare became over time a key part of an extraordinarily complicated political and economic world of American medicine. And throughout the whole period, 1966–99, Medicare's political fate was shaped as much by broader forces in the environment as by developments within its narrower medical care domain.

For example, in July 1976, Medicare had its tenth anniversary, but hardly anyone noticed. Attention then centered on the presidential race between Ford and Carter and, for American medicine, the leading topics were persistent medical inflation and the continuing, contentious dispute about national health insurance. In July 1986, Medicare marked its twentieth anniversary with considerable fanfare. National health insurance had fallen off the political agenda in the Reagan years, leaving Medicare a prominent object of attention (and, largely, affection). On Medicare's twenty-fifth birthday in 1991, the program faced severe financial pressures, as did American medicine generally, and nobody publicly celebrated its silver anniversary. By its thirtieth anniversary in 1996, Medicare was once again a major topic of American politics, the object of intense fiscal scrutiny by a Congress and a president negotiating the terms of a balanced budget that would emerge in the summer of 1997. At the century's close, Medicare returned to controversial status, the subject of a bipartisan commission that addressed, without agreement, whether the program required a transformative overhaul or incremental adjustment.

This story of Medicare's operational development is marked by both irony and turbulence. The social insurance philosophy that ensured its original appeal as a proposal used the trust fund terminology for Part A to suggest a sense of financial precommitment and thus stability to Medicare. But, over time, forecasts of the trust fund accounting—and projections of "insolvency"—undermined the very sense of security the trust fund was supposed to engender (Oberlander, 1995). The administrative compromises deemed necessary for Medicare's passage in 1965 nonetheless contributed to the subsequent and worrisome inflation in medical care. That development in turn produced effects quite inimical to the expansionist intentions of Medicare's original sponsors. The understanding of these discrepancies, surprises, and disappointments lies not so much in the Byzantine subtleties of legislative bargaining and the idiosyncrasies of political personalities as in the wider forces that framed this bargaining and shaped program operations after 1965.

7

Medicare's Politics: 1966–90

THE ORIGINS OF MEDICARE REVISITED

Medicare's complicated historical origins are difficult to explain in the quite different political environment of the 1990s. It is important, for example, to appreciate how peculiarly American the program is from an international perspective. No other industrial democracy now provides a separate compulsory health insurance program for its elderly citizens. None, moreover, began public health insurance with such a beneficiary group. Most other industrial democracies either started with coverage of parts of their workforce or, as in the case of Canada, incrementally expanded special programs for the poor to universal programs for one service (hospitals) and then to another (physicians) (Marmor, 1975). This contrast implies that distinctive American circumstances, rather than some common feature of modern societies, explain Medicare's programmatic birth.

Medicare's origins substantially determined both the initial design of the program and the expectations of how it was to develop over time. There is a tendency, particularly among those unfamiliar with the gestation of Medicare, to interpret its later difficulties as the product of initial stupidity in its design. The stupidity "thesis" goes as follows. If there are ways in which Medicare has failed to solve the problems of the elderly to which it was supposedly directed, it must be because those who enacted the law foolishly ignored the gap between the problems identified and the remedies offered. This view was vividly apparent, for example, in Ross Perot's comment, in his address to the National Press Club during the 1996 presidential campaign, that "none of our social programs," including Medicare, "were [sic] ever designed to work" (Perot, 1996).

The fact is that reformers in 1965 assumed hospitalization coverage was but the first step in Medicare's benefits and that more would follow under the same pattern of payroll financing as Social Security. Likewise, the strategy's proponents took for granted that eligibility would be gradually expanded to take in most, if not all, of the population, extending first perhaps to children and pregnant women. Medicare's promoters thought it obvious that the rhetoric of enactment should emphasize the expansion of access, not the regulation and reform of American medical care practices. The clear goal was to reduce the risks of financial disaster—for the elderly and their families—and the clear understanding in 1965 was that the Congress would demand a largely hands-off posture toward the doctors and hospitals providing the care Medicare would finance. Three decades and more after Medicare's enactment, that vision seems odd. It is now taken for granted that how one pays for medical care affects the care given. In the buildup to enactment in 1965, no such presumption existed.

As noted in Part I, the incremental strategy of the 1950s and early 1960s also assumed that Medicare's social insurance form was acceptable to the extent it sharply differentiated the program from the demeaning world of public assistance. "On welfare," in American parlance, is an expression that generally implies stigma, and Medicare's designers made certain the program's features put it firmly within the tradition of *"earned"* social-insurance benefits, not charitable dispensations. The initial program avoided a means test by restricting eligibility to persons over age 65 (and their spouses) who had contributed to the social security system during their working lives. Though shielded from the stigma of welfare, Medicare was unable, as we shall see, to escape from the growing problems of American medicine generally, especially medical inflation. Indeed the problem of cost control emerged as a largely unforeseen, recurring, and central influence on Medicare's development in the decades following its enactment. Instead of trying to expand Medicare's scope, reform efforts focused on containing Medicare's expenditures and rationalizing its administration. By the 1980s, the combination of persistent medical inflation and the increased popularity of anti-Washington rhetoric had for many commentators transformed the image of Medicare into an out-of-control entitlement.

THE POLITICS OF ACCOMMODATION:
MEDICARE'S IMPLEMENTATION AND SUBSEQUENT
EVOLUTION FROM 1966 TO 1970

Once under way, Medicare proved far more complex to administer than its parent pension programs within the Social Security Administration. Medicare expenditures varied with the use the elderly made of the program and with the charges and fees of medical providers. Technological changes in medicine increased costs unpredictably, whereas pension outlays were based on a rigid formula that related present benefits to past social-insurance payments. Medicare had to adapt to the behavior of both providers and beneficiaries. The Social Security pension program could largely focus on recipients and internal administration (Brown, 1985, 582). These differences in organizational tasks, coupled with Medicare's unexpected two-part insurance hybrid, produced a historically unprecedented level of complexity for Social Security's administrative elite.

Medicare's administrative arrangements reflected strong medical resistance to the program at the time of its enactment, as earlier chapters have emphasized. To hasten the program's implementation in the face of this resistance, Medicare's designers and initial administrators had sought a workable consensus in their negotiations with providers in the hospital, nursing home, and physician worlds. This willingness to accommodate explained the acceptance of benefit and payment policies that undoubtedly exerted inflationary pressure and certainly hindered the federal government's ability to control increases in the program's outlays. Elastic definitions of key legislative terms—particularly "reasonable costs" for hospitals and "customary charges" for physicians— proved to be significant loopholes that prompted energetic gaming strategies on the part of providers, as Chapter 5 notes. Unusual allowances for depreciation and capital costs—taken into account in determining reimbursement rates—contributed a built-in inflationary impetus. The use of private insurance companies as financial and administrative intermediaries initially provided an ideological and administrative buffer between the Social Security Administration and the world of American doctors and hospitals. But it also weakened government controls on the realities of reimbursement. It was left to these intermediaries, with long histories of close relations with providers, to determine administratively the reasonableness of costs under Part A and charges under Part B (Somers and Somers, 1967).

The truth is that in the early years of Medicare's implementation, the program's administrators were not organizationally disposed to confront most providers of medical services in ways necessary to restrain costs. SSA administrators prided themselves on their history of successful implementation of social insurance, and they needed the cooperation of all parties for Medicare's implementation to proceed as smoothly. Contentious efforts to clamp down on Medicare costs threatened this cooperative disposition. Medicare's designers, who were well aware of the argument for building inflation restraint into the program, were nonetheless reluctant to do so for fear of enraging Medicare providers (Feder, 1977, 23; Brown, 1985; Jacobs, 1993).

The late 1960s thus witnessed the efficient administration of a program whose design features were themselves inflationary. The results were predictable. Medicare expenditures swelled, as did the health budget of the nation as a whole. In the first year of Medicare's operation, as noted earlier, the average daily service charge in American hospitals increased by more than 20 percent. The average annual rate of expenditure growth over the next five years was 14 percent. Medicare's definition of "reasonable" charges paved the way for steep increases in physician fees. The rate of growth in physician fees more than doubled, from 3.8 percent in 1965 to 7.8 percent in 1966. The rate of increase in physician fees also remained high over the next five years, at 6.8 percent (Table 6.1), about twice the rate of inflation in the consumer price index (CPI) (Tables 7.1 and 7.2). Total Medicare reimbursements rose

Table 7.1. Annual Changes (%) in Physician Fees According to the Consumer Price Index for Fiscal Years 1967–71

Fiscal year	Physicians' fees (index, calendar year 1967 = 100)	Increase (%)
1967	96.9	7.4
1968	102.8	6.1
1969	109.1	6.1
1970	117.0	7.2
1971	125.8	7.5

Source: Howard West, "Five Years of Medicare—A Statistical Review," *Social Security Bulletin,* Dec. 1971, p. 21.

Table 7.2. Consumer Price Index and American Hospital Association Data for Hospital Expenses, Each Fiscal Year, 1967–71, and Annual Percentage Increases

Fiscal year	Hospital daily service charges		Hospital expenses per patient day (AHA)	
	Index (calendar year 1967 = 100)	Annual increase (%)	Amount	Annual increase (%)
1967	92.2	16.6	$53.67	12.5
1968	106.4	15.4	61.73	15.0
1969	120.5	13.3	70.13	13.6
1970	135.4	12.4	80.71	15.1
1971	152.8	12.9	91.37	13.2

Source: Data for daily service charges are from the *Consumer Price Index,* Bureau of Labor Statistics; data for hospital expenses per patient day are from "Hospital Indicators," *Hospitals,* Journal of the American Hospital Association. (From Howard West, "Five Years of Medicare—A Statistical Review," *Social Security Bulletin,* Dec. 1971, p. 21.)

72 percent, from $4.6 billion in 1967 to $7.9 billion in 1971 (see Figure 7.1; Gornick et al., 1985, 43, Table 25). Over the same period (Figure 7.1), the number of Medicare enrollees rose only 6 percent, from 19.5 million in 1967 to 20.7 million in 1971 (ibid., 36, Table 17).

With the full benefit of hindsight, it is easy to criticize the accommodationist posture of Medicare's initial administrators. At the time of the program's enactment, however, Medicare's legislative mandate was to protect the nation's elderly from the economic burden of illness *without* significantly interfering with the traditional organization of American medicine. It was with this aim in mind that Medicare's first administrators sought an accommodation to ensure a smooth, speedy start for the program. Not until later did Medicare come to be seen as a powerful means to constrain both the costs and practices of American medicine (Ball, 1972, 47–48; Marmor, 1987, 43).

THE 1970s: INEFFECTUAL REFORMS AND INTERMITTENT PROGRESS

By 1970, there was a bipartisan consensus that the United States faced what amounted to a crisis in the costs of medical care (U.S. Senate, Committee on Finance, 1970). Though partly stimulated by Medicare's rapidly rising expenditures, health policy initiatives in the early 1970s in fact concentrated on reforming American medicine overall, not revamping Medicare. The sense of crisis spawned two separate lines of policy development aimed at controlling medical costs.

The first line of development constituted a reawakening of the movement for national health insurance. This effort reached its apex in the 1974 competition over which plan—Nixon's Comprehensive Health Insurance Plan (CHIP), the Kennedy-Mills bill, or the Long-Ribicoff catastrophic scheme—would pass (Feder, Holahan, and Marmor, 1980). In that political context, the reform of Medicare was subordinated to grander designs.

The second line of policy development consisted of more limited, fragmentary initiatives that addressed the conventional topics of health policy and management (quality, capital spending, and planning). Originating outside Medicare's administration (and, in fact, viewed with hostility by some Medicare administrators), the new programs relied on state and local activity and were intended to circumvent the "protectiveness and particularism" of program specialists (Brown, 1985, 589). For example, the Social Security Amendments of 1972 (P.L. 92603) established professional standards review organizations (PSROs) to review the care received by federally funded patients; encouraged use of health maintenance organizations (HMOs) in Medicare; required states

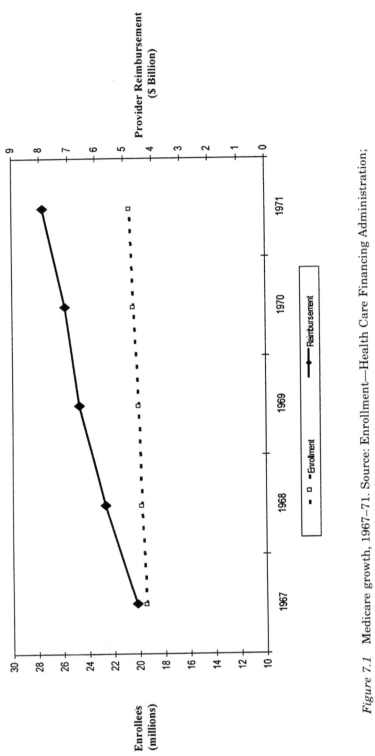

Figure 7.1 Medicare growth, 1967–71. Source: Enrollment—Health Care Financing Administration; reimbursement—Gornick et al. (1985).

to review capital-spending projects for hospitals; and authorized federal support for state experiments with prospective-payment systems. In 1974, Congress enacted the Health Planning and Resources Development Act (P.L. 93641), which created more than 200 health systems agencies (HSAs) to oversee areawide medical planning across the nation.

These fragmented measures were part of a broader national health insurance strategy that ultimately failed to materialize (Morone and Marmor, 1981, 431–50). When national health insurance failed to pass Congress, the other planning and regulatory programs were left without the full force of the financing national health insurance would have provided. They became incomplete alternatives to comprehensive reform and, because of their contribution to the diffusion of federal authority, stood in the way of centralized reform later (Brown, 1985, 587; Marmor, 1990, 33). These partial reforms, one sees in retrospect, were inadequate measures for controlling medical costs. They left the basic inflationary structure of the medical care industry—retrospective payment, pluralistic financing, and intermediary administration—largely intact.

The adoption of these fragmentary measures did, however, reveal two important features of health politics in the United States that are critical for understanding how Medicare developed administratively over time. First, no matter how large the public subsidies and how substantial the public interest in the distribution, financing, and quality of services dominated by private actors, the American impulse is to disperse authority, finance, and control. In an industry like medical care, this reluctance to consolidate authority is a recipe for inflation, as the past three decades, as well as ample international experience, demonstrate (White, 1995; Evans, Barer, and Hertzman, 1991; Marmor, 1976). Second, the initiatives of the early 1970s illustrate the adherence of federal policymakers to a theory of medical care that had slowly emerged throughout the post–World War II period. This widely held view, sometimes referred to as hierarchical regionalism, presumed that "more medical care for individuals distributed by regional hierarchies [of providers] would lead to better health for populations" (Fox, 1986, 208). On the basis of that conviction, governments acted to subsidize "research and professional education, increase the supply of professionals and facilities, establish and encourage regional hierarchies [of hospitals], and reduce the direct costs of care to patients" (ibid.).

As the prospects for national health insurance faded in the last half of the 1970s, legislative interest shifted from new programs consistent with national health insurance to a renewed emphasis on cost control itself. By the end of the decade, though, there was little progress on the anti-inflation front either.

The 1972 Social Security Amendments and the 1973 federal legislation supporting so-called health maintenance organizations (HMOs)
marked the beginning of flirtation with market-based versions of cost
control. HMOs, first called prepaid group practices, were identified with
the left wing of American medical reform from the 1930s to the early
1970s. The prepaid group practice model was associated with the ideal
of universal insurance, the appeal of capitative payment, and the conviction that nonprofit forms of organization were superior. HMOs in the
1970s represented a largely Republican repackaging (and transformation) of the early largely Democratic model. The reform in the 1970s was
an effort to find an apparently bipartisan solution to the nation's medical inflation problem (Brown, 1983). By reversing the inflationary
incentives of fee-for-service medicine, HMOs were expected to use capitation payment, to enhance competition in the delivery and price of medical care, and thereby to reduce costs. Advocates—sometimes labeled
"public entrepreneurs"—made heady predictions about the speed with
which HMOs would come to dominate and thus reform American medicine (Oliver, 1996; Brown, 1983).

The expansion of HMOs in the 1970s, however, did not live up to the
inflated predictions; the growth of membership was modest throughout
the 1970s (see Figure 7.2), while national medical expenditures continued to rise sharply (Figure 7.2). Federal efforts to use HMOs as the key
instrument of cost containment, according to most analysts, were a tale
of failure (Brown, 1983).

The Carter administration, genuinely alarmed by rising hospital
costs, concluded that "clearly, the time ha[d] come—indeed it has been
here for a long time—to bite the bullet on hospital costs" (Mondale,
1978, 67). The Carter administration's attempts to secure passage of
legislation that explicitly regulated hospital costs was blocked. But
federal efforts to regulate the hospital industry did put it on the
defensive. The industry subsequently adopted a "voluntary effort" to
control spending, one that also disappointed in practice (Peterson,
1995).

In 1977 a new Health Care Financing Administration (HCFA) was
created within HEW to administer both Medicare and Medicaid. This
pulled Medicare away from the Social Security Administration's managerial ethos and bureaucratic style. Medicare became "one element in
the broader universe of federal health care financing programs," rather
than a freestanding component of the nation's social-insurance system
(Brown, 1985, 591). With this change, Medicare administrators within
HCFA became more concerned with the financing of health services
than with social insurance. This change would, over time, prove to be
critical to altering not only the practical administration but also the

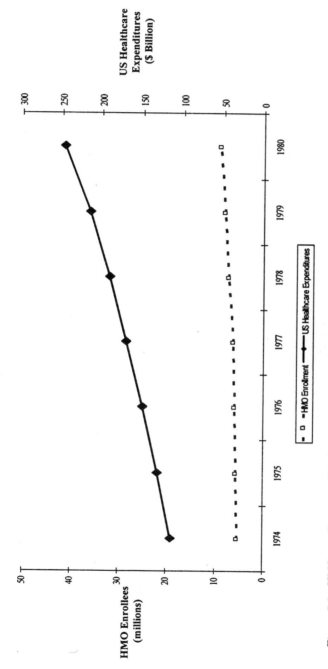

Figure 7.2 HMO enrollment *vs.* U.S. healthcare expenditures, 1974–80. Source: enrollment—National HMO Census, 1981, Department of Health and Human Services; expenditures—Office of National Statistics, HCFA.

politics of Medicare. Congress also enacted in 1977 the Medicaid Anti-Fraud and Abuse Amendments (P.L. 95142), legislation that charged HCFA with collecting and analyzing hospital cost data. These seemingly technical changes and the shift in administrative outlook accompanying HCFA's establishment were more important than they appeared. They prepared the way, among other things, for the 1983 reform of Medicare's method of paying hospitals on a prospective basis (Oberlander, 1995).

By the end of the decade, the piecemeal reforms of the early 1970s were in disarray. From one side came charges that such fragmented measures had predictably failed to restrain inflation in the health industry. From the other side came criticism that piecemeal change had left 30 million or more American citizens uninsured for the expenses of illness and both Medicare and Medicaid in precarious financial condition. Medicare's administrative divorce from social security in the late 1970s did, it is true, prompt hope for the program's reform. Nonetheless, this administrative shift distracted attention from the need for more substantial policy reforms that would address the fundamental sources of medical inflation, the erosion of Medicare's benefits, and the confusion experienced by its beneficiaries.

Largely unreconstructed in benefits and cost control instruments, Medicare continued to experience large annual increases in expenditures as the 1970s came to a close. "By 1980, Medicare was the second largest domestic program and the fastest growing" (Moon, 1993, 41). Nevertheless, because it was still widely viewed and supported as social insurance, Medicare escaped severe budget cuts. Increases in Medicare spending contributed to the much larger problem of recurrent annual increases in overall health spending. Claims of strain were fully justified. The growth of expenditures on medical care far exceeded the rate of inflation in the general economy throughout most of the 1970s with the result that medical-care spending constituted an ever increasing proportion of the gross national product (GNP), rising from 7.1 percent in 1970 to 8.9 percent in 1980 (see Figure 7.3). Medicare, and all of medical care, was consuming a larger and larger piece of the economic pie, crowding out spending on other goods and services.

Despite the rapid growth of Medicare expenditures, however, the elderly actually experienced significant erosion in their program benefits. By the mid-1980s, the nation's senior citizens were spending the same proportion of their incomes on medical care as they had before Medicare's enactment (see Figure 7.4) (Schlesinger and Drumheller, 1988).

The Medicare program also produced considerable confusion for elderly citizens that persisted and, some would argue, worsened over time.

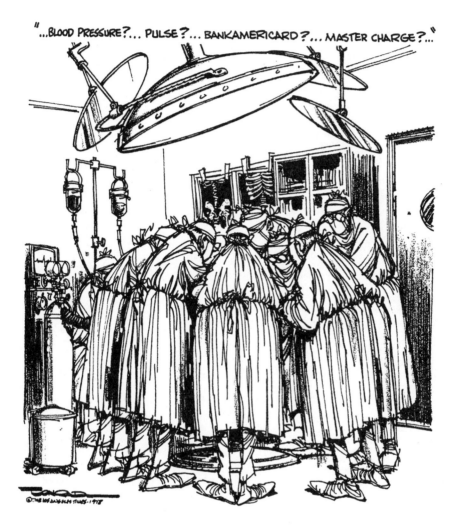

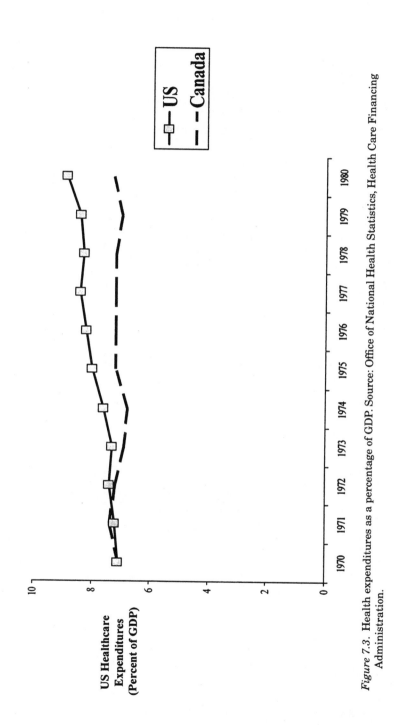

Figure 7.3 Health expenditures as a percentage of GDP. Source: Office of National Health Statistics, Health Care Financing Administration.

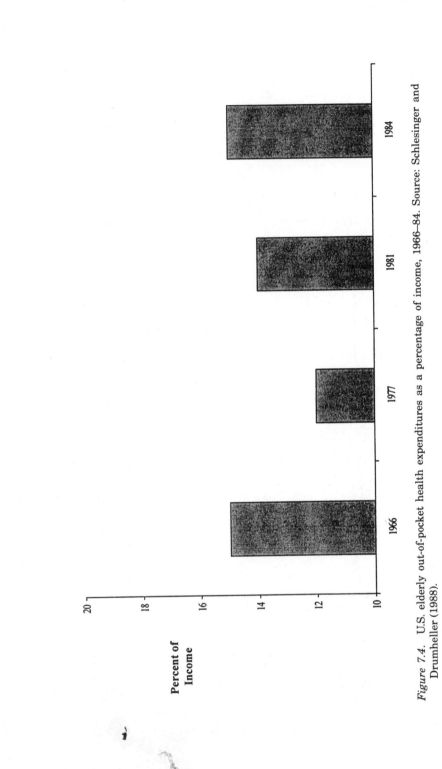

Figure 7.4. U.S. elderly out-of-pocket health expenditures as a percentage of income, 1966–84. Source: Schlesinger and Drumheller (1988).

The separate coverage of hospital and physician services, borrowed wholesale from the conventional Blue Cross and Blue Shield plans of the period, was easy enough for the Congress to stitch together in the bargaining of 1965. For the elderly, though, it meant two different programs, each with its own financing sources, its own fiscal intermediary, and different deductibles, coinsurance provisions, and forms. Part A financing came from earmarked deductions from wages (the health insurance component of FICA contributions); Part B drew its financing from both individual monthly premiums and general tax revenues. To this mix was added a third level of complexity with supplementary policies sold by major commercial and nonprofit health insurers, the so-called Medigap plans. Since these supplementary policies took Medicare's benefits as their baseline, Medigap benefits were typically expressed by reference to the elements not covered or only partially covered by Medicare's Parts A and B.

What was initially confusing became more complicated with time and administrative changes. With the shift of Medicare to HCFA, Social Security offices throughout the country ceased to regard Medicare's administrative matters as their business. For the elderly, this change meant less assistance with the delays, complicated documents, and requests for clarification that from the beginning of Medicare had come from SSA offices. Beneficiaries were now left to cope with this administrative maze largely on their own; their link to Medicare was the toll-free telephone numbers of the insurance companies that act as the program's fiscal intermediaries. It is this confusion that constituted an important legacy of both the incremental strategy of Medicare's founders and the subsequent administrative adjustments made during the 1970s in the hopes of successful cost containment and tidier federal administration of both Medicare and Medicaid (Oberlander, 1995).

THE 1980s: THE CHALLENGE OF THE REAGAN ERA

Medicare, after nearly fifteen years of relatively quiet controversy in the specialized politics of medical care finance, acquired much greater political salience in the Reagan era. Always of great interest to those in the medical world, Medicare was a second-order topic in the mass politics of the late 1960s and the 1970s. The oil crisis of the 1973–74 period and the consequent "stagflation" had joined with Social Security finance as the high-priority items on the national public-policy agenda. This is not to say that Medicare's politics had been uneventful. Rather, it is simply that Medicare had faced ordinary interest group politics, specially protected under the mantle of social insurance's entitlement theories and the elderly's reputed political influence. That protected status was what the 1980s were to challenge.

The challenge came in two forms. The first was inclusion of Medicare cutbacks in the grand design of the Reagan fiscal policy of 1981. The second was the bold departure in Medicare's reimbursement policy that the DRG (diagnosis-related group) reform of 1983 represented.

The Reagan administration came to power brandishing anti-welfare-state and antiregulatory rhetoric. It promised to reduce, not expand, the role of the federal government in the domestic sphere. The administration, like others, lamented the relentlessness of medical inflation and the budget implications of Medicare's rapidly increasing expenditures. But the administration approached cost control from a distinctive viewpoint. It was preoccupied with restraining the costs of public programs, not with reducing medical inflation per se. This preoccupation meant that Medicare policy increasingly became budget reduction politics.

When taken together, the Reagan administration's health policies emphasized four themes: reducing the federal medical care budget; restraining payments to Medicare providers; cutting benefits, in particular through increased cost-sharing for Medicare and Medicaid recipients; and claiming that excessive health insurance causes medical inflation (Marmor, 1988).

Though central to the Reagan administration's policy initiatives, the theory that "excessive" health insurance causes medical inflation and the overutilization of medical services was open to serious question. The evidence is clear that increased utilization itself has played a small role in driving up Medicare's costs (Freeland and Schendler, 1984; Moon, 1993, 42–43, Table 3.1). The theory also overlooked the crucial role of providers—especially in fee-for-service practice—in fueling medical inflation. In addition, the commitment to cost-sharing as the central medical-inflation remedy had a fundamental flaw: relative indifference to the degree to which cost-sharing discourages early diagnosis, shifts costs to the sick, and is not a necessary feature of effective cost control (Evans, Barer, and Stoddart, 1994; Conrad and Marmor, 1983).

The Reagan administration's efforts to restrict payments to providers—the enactment of prospective hospital payment legislation (DRGs) in 1983 and of a new fee schedule for physicians (Resource-Based Relative Value Scale, "RBRVS") in 1989—were much more effective in achieving the overarching goal of restraining the growth of Medicare expenditures. Indeed, these two payment measures were the most significant developments in Medicare policy since the program's inception. The reform of Medicare's methods of paying hospitals and doctors reshaped the program's politics, introducing what amounted to a new regulatory regime (Oberlander, 1995).

Frustrated by the hospital industry's failure to maintain their so-called voluntary effort to control costs, and concerned over the impact of rising expenditures on Medicare's trust fund, Congress quickly adopted the administration's prospective hospital payment method for the program (Smith, 1992). Under this form of payment, based on diagnosis-related groups (the DRGs with which New Jersey had experimented for some years), the Medicare program set out to pay fixed prospective rates for specific diagnoses (for example, angina pectoris or simple pneumonia). By introducing these new elements—*pro*spective rather than retrospective payment, and fixed rates based on diagnostic categories rather than reimbursement of costs incurred—DRGs provided the administration with a powerful tool to pursue its budgetary objectives.

Two features distinguished this new regime of requiring prospective payment to hospitals. First, it embodied a clearly technocratic approach to containing the costs of medical care. The technical garb served, as discussed later in this chapter, to keep disputes over cost control out of the political process. Second, it allowed the federal government to exert far more influence over reimbursement to Medicare providers than it had previously employed. DRG reimbursement is really a sophisticated form of government price controls. Prospective rates change the incentives facing hospitals by replacing cost reimbursement with a fixed payment per diagnosis, one that reflects average costs in a medical market. Hospitals whose costs exceeded the DRG payment were expected to absorb the loss, and those whose costs fell below the fixed payment could keep the savings. In this manner, DRGs were expected to encourage more efficient provision of medical care by making hospitals responsible for the financial consequences of their practices.

There were, critics claimed at the time, major dangers of this much-heralded policy innovation. First, restricting prospective rates to Medicare patients alone created some incentive for hospitals to shift costs to privately financed patients. (Cost shifting by hospitals, to the extent it occurred, would reduce Medicare's expenditures, but not medical inflation.) Second, to the degree that hospitals were unable to shift Medicare's costs to other payers, Medicare patients would become less welcome. As a result, the elderly's access to hospitals—or extended stays—would be restricted as Medicare's prospective payments to the nation's hospitals tightened. The problem of restricted access would be most severe for the sickest patients with the most complex medical problems. Restrictive payments by Medicaid had by this period already reduced the access to medical care of many of the poor (Lurie et al., 1984). Third, even efficient hospitals would face financial jeopardy if they served large numbers of government-financed patients. These fears notwithstanding, DRGs did prove to be an effective means of

reducing the ongoing inflation in hospital costs under Medicare, helping the Reagan administration to contain the size of the federal medical care budget. From 1985 to 1990, hospital expenditures under
Medicare dropped from 28.9 to 26.1 percent of total national hospital
expenditures (Letsch et al., 1992, Table 17), a sign that federal interventions are capable of bringing Medicare expenditures under control.
Medicare's per capita expenditures grew less rapidly than those of private insurance (on services that were provided by both) from 1984 to
1992 (see Figure 7.5).

One cannot discuss Medicare in the 1980s without reference to the
passage and subsequent repeal of the Medicare Catastrophic Coverage
Act of 1988 (MCCA). The story of the MCCA is particularly instructive
in one respect. It highlights the connection between Medicare's interest
group politics and the new politics of deficit reduction. In a striking
deviation from the Reagan administration's efforts to restrict expenditures, the MCCA greatly expanded Medicare's benefits. Rather than
reflecting the ideology of the Reagan administration, however, the legislation was largely the work of a single individual, Otis Bowen. The
1982 National Commission on Social Security Reform, under Bowen's
leadership, had recommended that Medicare hospitalization coverage
be expanded to an unlimited number of days, that its hospital and
skilled-nursing-facility coinsurance requirements be eliminated, and
that Medicare beneficiaries be offered an optional Part B benefit (physician services), one that would put a cap on out-of-pocket expenses. It
was these recommendations that Bowen, when he subsequently became secretary of Health and Human Services under President Reagan, sought to enact (Oberlander, 1995).

Bowen's efforts to promote catastrophic-care coverage tapped into a
widespread dissatisfaction, especially among Democrats in Congress,
with Medicare's limited coverage of care for chronic conditions (Rovner,
1987). The new benefits under the Catastrophic Coverage Act were
quite extensive. They included not just those of the 1982 National Commission, but also expanded provisions for hospice care, home health
services, mammography screening, outpatient prescription drugs,
guaranteed payment of Medicare premiums for the impoverished elderly, and protection against the impoverishment of a spouse from nursing home expenses.[1] The legislation did not include, however, what was
perhaps the most important benefit sought by the elderly and seen by
them as a central feature of catastrophic protection: namely, the coverage of long-term institutionalization in nursing homes.

The method chosen to finance this expansion of benefits was, in
equal parts, a product of political necessity and historical accident.
Reflecting his commitment to reduce the federal budget for medical

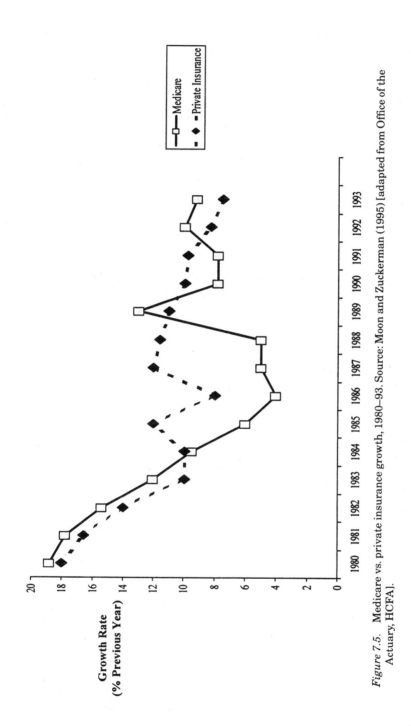

Figure 7.5. Medicare vs. private insurance growth, 1980–93. Source: Moon and Zuckerman (1995) [adapted from Office of the Actuary, HCFA].

care, President Reagan had agreed to support the legislation only on condition that it add nothing to the federal deficit. The remaining options for financing the benefits package were limited, however. With the Social Security payroll tax already at what was then considered a politically acceptable maximum, and with general tax increases regarded as infeasible, the only available alternative was to have the elderly finance this coverage themselves. The means was an anomalous increase in the monthly Part B premiums paid by beneficiaries. Though these premiums had continued to be earmarked for physician services ever since Medicare's enactment, the legislation mandated that the increased premium be used for hospital and other care historically funded exclusively by payroll taxes. In an additional departure from historical practice, the legislation required a subgroup of beneficiaries—the more affluent elderly—to pay a supplemental premium, with a limit of $800 in 1989.

The sharpest criticism of the new Catastrophic Coverage Act came from some elderly groups themselves. Here, again, the origins and evolution of Medicare played an important role in the politics of the legislation—in this case by framing the elderly's response to both its substance and method of financing. In providing coverage for extended hospitalizations rather than long-term institutionalized care, the legislation addressed a problem experienced by few of the elderly and left unaddressed a "catastrophic" situation dreaded by many. This failure was, in itself, sufficient to guarantee no more than a lukewarm response. Much more importantly, the legislation encountered especially strong opposition among the affluent elderly. The act's highly progressive tax burden fell most heavily on this group, but they were, in fact, least likely to need its coverage. Many among this group already possessed supplemental insurance—often financed by their former employers. This group was capable, moreover, of organizing a political effort—indeed, a revolt—against the "reform."

In a strategy that took advantage of the chronic misunderstandings and confusions plaguing Medicare beneficiaries from the inception of the program, elderly groups such as the National Committee to Preserve Social Security and Medicare succeeded in conveying the impression that all of the elderly—not just the most affluent—would be burdened by the extra premium. The intensity of the opposition to MCCA was captured by a widely disseminated photograph of Chairman of Ways and Means Dan Rostenkowski (D., Ill.) being chased into his car by angry, sign-waving senior citizens (Himelfarb, 1995). A year and a half after the Catastrophic Coverage Act was resoundingly enacted, it was even more resoundingly repealed. Ironically, the historical failure of Medicare to provide complete medical coverage for the elderly had itself created the demand for the supplemental insurance we call Medigap plans. The possession of Medigap insurance in turn motivated the affluent elderly to oppose an act providing just such expanded coverage to all Medicare beneficiaries.[2]

Politically criticized for a well-intended effort to expand Medicare benefits, Congress returned with enthusiasm to the technical tasks of making regulatory adjustments in Medicare that would reduce program expenditures. While repealing the Catastrophic Coverage Act, the Congress added two new components to a regulatory structure, initiated with DRGs, designed to restrict payments to providers: a revamped physician fee schedule (RBRVS) and direct controls on the volume of physician services, the so-called volume performance standards. Like the prospective payment to hospitals, the fee schedule utilized a complex technical methodology to change Medicare's mode of paying doctors. Formally known as the Resource-Based Relative Value Scale (RBRVS), the method calculated the fee for a given service by estimating the time, training, and skill necessary to perform it.

The impetus for physician payment reform was the continuing, substantial increases in Medicare Part B expenditures. Throughout the 1980s, Congress had enacted a series of incremental measures designed to curb the program's payments to doctors. From 1984 to 1986, for example, Medicare imposed a two-and-a-half-year freeze on Medicare physician fees. Despite the freeze, Medicare's physician bill continued to climb. Rising by an annual average rate of 11.6 percent during this period (Rovner, 1987), Medicare's physician payments reflected increases in the volume of services provided as well as the transfer of many inpatient hospital activities to ambulatory settings not subject to prospective payment (see Figure 7.6) (Oliver, 1993). In this context, the goal of the RBRVS fee schedule was to restrain costs by rewarding less expensive primary care and by reducing the rewards of costly surgical and diagnostic procedures. The volume performance standards sought to hold down costs by constraining the escalating volume of physician services.

Both the prospective payment arrangements for hospitals and the new physician fee schedule were examples of what Larry Brown has rightly called "technocratic corporatism." They involved complex formulas for pricing medical services, accompanied by government-provider negotiations over the details of the reimbursement schemes (Brown, 1985). To the extent that these cost control initiatives relied on such technical complexities, they conformed with an American tendency to try to avoid (or at least mask) explicitly conflictual political decisions (Morone, 1994). Implicitly, however, these initiatives were deeply political in character. And despite their guise of technical neu-

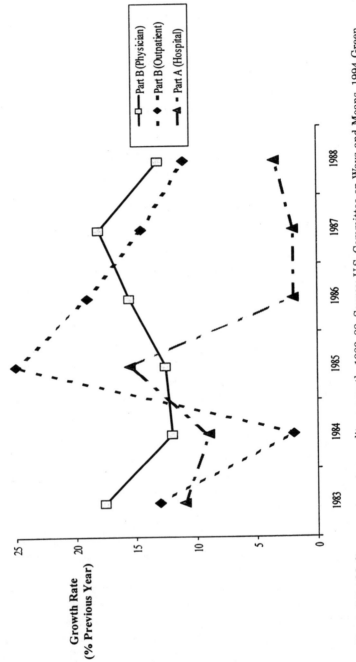

Figure 7.6. Medicare component expenditure growth, 1983–88. Source: U.S. Committee on Ways and Means, 1994 Green Book; Medicare Payment Advisory Commission.

trality and objectivity, they generated considerable dissatisfaction and conflict, especially within the medical profession. For example, the decision to reallocate funds in favor of primary care practitioners, rather than simply limit compensation across the board, set up tension between specialized physicians and primary care physicians. By dividing physicians, these seemingly technical changes moved part of the battle from one between organized medicine and the government, to one within the medical profession, a shift that was to have implications for the future of Medicare.

CONCLUSION

The politics of Medicare in the 1980s we have sketched are unintelligible, however, if viewed simply as technical policy adjustments in an era of fiscal strain. The changes arose as much from more general shifts in the political environment as from technical considerations of reimbursement. On the one hand, the combination of increased defense spending and sharply reduced tax revenues had put all social spending in a political vise. Social Security escaped that vise through the legislative changes in 1983 (which brought the program's finances into balance) and the subsequent insulation from the automatic spending reductions of the 1985 Gramm-Rudman legislation (Ball, 1988). Medicare remained within the vulnerable set of programs for the rest of the 1980s and beyond.

On the other hand, the world of American medicine was very different—politically and institutionally—from what it had been at Medicare's enactment. No one of political significance advocated universal health insurance in the 1980s. The deficits of the Reagan (and Bush) administrations dominated political discourse and set severe limits on what seemed sensible to discuss in any social welfare program, including medical care. The policy debate was shaped as well by the debris from the reform disappointments of the 1970s and by the frustrated expansionary expectations of Medicare's early promoters. In that environment of the 1980s, celebrators of market reform in medicine had an unusually powerful effect, offering the prospect of more services at less cost, with less involvement by the government (Marmor, Boyer, and Greenberg, 1983).

Attracted by the gold mine of funds flowing through a system of retrospective, cost-based reimbursement, the captains of American capitalism had come to see opportunity in the 1970s where politicians had found causes for complaint (Marmor, Schlesinger, and Smithey, 1986). In the hospital world, small chains of for-profit companies—the

Humanas and the Hospital Corporations of America, to name the most prominent examples—grew into large corporations during the disappointing regulatory decade of the 1970s. Industrial giants, like Baxter-Travenol and American Hospital Supply, took their conventional plans for competitive growth and extended them through vertical and horizontal integration. Although this economic concentration increased the power of the health care industry, it simultaneously contributed to a decline in the power of medicine as a profession. The power of the medical profession was waning for a variety of reasons: a glut of physicians leaving medical school, the rise of importance of insurance companies as arbiters of what care would be covered, the disillusionment with the AMA as a dispassionate guardian of the nation's health, increasing friction between general care physicians and specialists—aggravated by the late 1980s RBRVS physician fee scale, as well as the move to more centralized and bureaucratic systems of "integrated health care."

All these changes in the structure of American medicine took place within the context of increasingly antiregulatory and anti-Washington rhetoric. Both Democratic and Republican elites were influenced by a generation of policy analysts, mostly economists, who ridiculed both the costliness and the captured quality of the decisions made by independent regulatory agencies in Washington. The Civil Aeronautics Board and the airlines industry came to symbolize the distortions likely when government regulates industry; and, with time, the convention of describing any set of related activities with economic significance as an "industry" demythologized medicine as well (Derthick and Quirk, 1995).[3] So, even before the Reagan administration took office, the political environment was receptive to the celebration of "competitive forces" in medical care, for getting government off the back of the American medical establishment, and for letting the fresh air of deregulation solve the problems of access, cost, and quality.

Given this setting, it is a deep irony that the most consequential health-policy innovation of the Reagan period—Medicare's prospective payment method of DRGs—was an exceedingly sophisticated, highly regulatory form of administered prices. The further irony is that the rate of medical inflation somewhat declined (see Figure 7.7 for 1983 and 1984 statistics) at precisely the period when the growing federal deficit made unthinkable a direct attack on the problem of the uninsured, let alone reforms to improve the scope of Medicare's benefits.

The momentum for market-based reform was ultimately slowed by the conflict between the Reagan administration's ideology and its short-term priorities in health policy. Competition appealed to the administration's preference for the use of market devices in public policy. Nonetheless, the administration's determination to contain federal expenditures made the speedy reduction of Medicare's costs an urgent

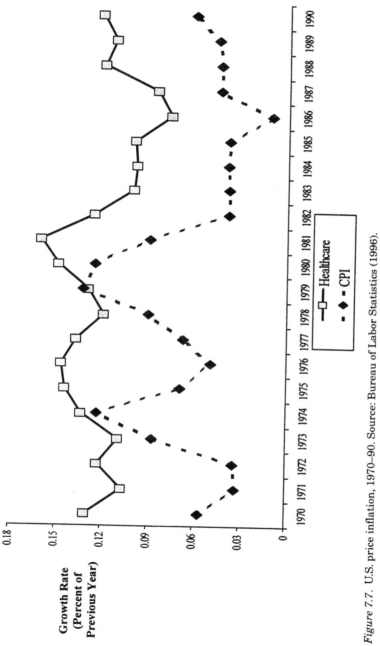

Figure 7.7. U.S. price inflation, 1970–90. Source: Bureau of Labor Statistics (1996).

priority. Making medical-care markets more competitive was not a plausible strategy to satisfy short-term fiscal goals (Marmor and Christianson, 1982). Restraining health costs through market reform requires precipitating an organizational revolution in the delivery and governance of medical services. And from the Reagan administration's perspective, this revolution could not be carried out with sufficient speed. It was at best a long-range strategy that would have no impact on current federal health expenditures. The only option was to disregard the Reagan administration's ideological commitment to competition, and to embark on a course of strict regulation and direct control of payments to providers.

By the early 1980s, the difficulties of Medicare had become those of American medicine in general, rather than of the program alone. The remedial proposals enacted during that decade were, of necessity, substantially broader than the tinkering needed to address problems with Social Security's cash programs (Light, 1986; Marmor and Mashaw, 1988). The politics of Medicare thus diverged from those of retirement and disability pensions. This divergence was the consequence not only of differences in administering a program of third-party payment instead of pension checks, but also of the rapid pace of change in the world of modern American medicine, and of the continued strain of medical inflation. As a result, Medicare became more vulnerable to a major legislative intervention than other parts of the nation's social-insurance system. A particularly important change was Medicare's administrative relocation to HCFA in the late 1970s. That seemingly innocent shift further separated Medicare from the social-insurance roots that had given it its initial legitimacy, defined its goals, and linked it locally to elderly beneficiaries. At the same time, the politics of budget deficits, relentless medical inflation, and America's presumed aversion to tax increases made an expansion of Medicare highly unlikely.

This situation presented both opportunities and risks by the end of the 1980s. The very unsettled state of Medicare policy offered the chance to rediscover the reasons why the nation had agreed in 1965 that medical care for the elderly should be especially protected from the influence of personal wealth and the randomness of illness and injury. Moreover, there is always the possibility in medical care that better allocation of existing funds could lead to more appropriate care without necessarily paying more. Unlike pensions, where increased benefits would necessarily entail higher outlays, the reallocation of funds freed up by reduced payments for unnecessary or harmful medical care might be able to cover expanded benefits.

But with opportunities came risks. Many policy suggestions could worsen the circumstances of older citizens in the name of competition, rationalization, and reform. Cost containment could easily lead to the withdrawal of needed care. Indeed, there were numerous examples after 1983 of cases in which DRGs' financial incentives induced hospitals to discharge older patients prematurely. Cost containment—when applied to Medicare alone—could simply shift costs to others or make Medicare patients less welcome as patients. Providing Medicare beneficiaries with vouchers for HMOs might as easily prompt providers to search for the healthier old ("cream skimming") as a result in the provision of more efficient medical care to *all* beneficiaries. Finally, the focus on budgetary aggregates driven by deficit politics could well obscure the reality that despite Medicare's expenditures of $130 billion in 1991, millions of older Americans remained without effective protection from the catastrophic financial consequences of chronic illness. The mantle of social insurance, so crucial to Medicare's origins, by the late 1980s provided no certainty of protection from these risks.

NOTES

1. Prescription drug coverage, which did not play a large role in the public debate over the legislation, would prove important in the legislation's subsequent repeal. After the bill's enactment, updated prescription drug usage figures caused a substantial increase in the estimated cost of the MCCA prescription drug benefit. That in turn led congressional deficit hawks to join the calls for repeal (Moon, 1996, 132–33). Once again, deficit politics played a role in Medicare's politics.

2. By the time of MCCA's repeal, opposition to the act was widespread among all elderly, and went well beyond the efforts of any particular group (Himelfarb, 1995, 79). As noted by Richard Himelfarb in his detailed postmortem of MCCA, the *perception* of Medicare beneficiaries (inaccurate in many cases) that the MCCA would increase their Medicare premiums in order to duplicate benefits they were already paying for was highly influential in their decision to oppose the act (Himelfarb, 1995, 71).

3. The rise of for-profit chains and health care industrial corporations lent credence to the notion that medicine could and should be treated more like an industry and less like a profession. In addition to the general antiregulatory tone, there was growing support for devolving any regulation to a lower level, be it regional, state or local, which, in theory, would be more sensitive and sensible.

MEDICARE HOSPITAL INSURANCE (PART A) COVERED SERVICES FOR 1997

Services	Benefit	Medicare Pays	You Pay
HOSPITALIZATION Semiprivate room and board, general nursing and other hospital services and supplies. (Medicare payments based on benefit periods; see pg. 10.)	First 60 days	All but $760	$760
	61st to 90th day	All but $190 a day	$190 a day
	91st to 150th day*	All but $380 a day	$380 a day
	Beyond 150 days	Nothing	All costs
SKILLED NURSING FACILITY CARE Semiprivate room and board, skilled nursing and rehabilitative services, and other services and supplies. **	First 20 days	100% of approved amount	Nothing
	Additional 80 days	All but $95 a day	Up to $95 a day
	Beyond 100 days	Nothing	All costs
HOME HEALTH CARE Part-time or intermittent skilled care, home health aide services, durable medical equipment and supplies, and other services.	Unlimited as long as you meet Medicare requirements for home health care benefits.	100% of approved amount for services; 80% of approved amount for durable medical equipment.	Nothing for services; 20% of approved amount for durable medical equipment.
HOSPICE CARE Pain relief, symptom management, and support services for the terminally ill.	For as long as doctor certifies need.	All but limited costs for outpatient drugs and inpatient respite care.	Limited cost sharing for outpatient drugs and inpatient respite care.
BLOOD When furnished by a hospital or skilled nursing facility during a covered stay.	Unlimited during a benefit period if medically necessary.	All but first 3 pints per calendar year.	For first 3 pints.***

    * 60 reserve days may be used only once.
  ** Neither Medicare nor Medigap insurance will pay for most nursing home care.
*** To the extent the three pints of blood are paid for or replaced under one part of Medicare during the calendar year, they do not have to be paid for or replaced under the other part.

1997 Part A monthly premium: $311 with fewer than 30 quarters of Medicare-covered employment; $187 with 30 or more quarters, but fewer than 40 quarters of covered employment. Most beneficiaries do not have to pay a premium for Part A.

 Medicare Handbook

MEDICARE MEDICAL INSURANCE (PART B) COVERED SERVICES FOR 1997

Services	Benefit	Medicare Pays	You Pay
MEDICAL EXPENSES Physician's services, inpatient and outpatient medical and surgical services and supplies, physical, occupational and speech therapy, diagnostic tests, and durable medical equipment.	Unlimited services if medically necessary, except for the services of independent physical and occupational therapists.	80% of approved amount (after $100 deductible); 50% of approved amount for most outpatient mental health services; up to $720 a year each for independent physical and occupational therapy.	$100 deductible;* 20% of approved amount after deductible; charges above approved amount;** 50% for most outpatient mental health services; 20% of first $900 for each independent physical and occupational therapy and all charges thereafter each year.
CLINICAL LABORATORY SERVICES Blood tests, urinalysis, and more.	Unlimited if medically necessary.	Generally 100% of approved amount.	Nothing for services.
HOME HEALTH CARE*** Part-time or intermittent skilled care, home health aide services, durable medical equipment and supplies and other services.	Unlimited as long as you meet Medicare requirements.	100% of approved amount for services; 80% of approved amount for durable medical equipment.	Nothing for services; 20% of amount approved for durable medical equipment.
OUTPATIENT HOSPITAL SERVICES Services for the diagnosis or treatment of an illness or injury.	Unlimited if medically necessary.	Medicare payment to hospital based on hospital costs.	20% of whatever the hospital charges (after $100 deductible).*
BLOOD	Unlimited if medically necessary.	80% of approved amount (after $100 deductible and starting with 4th pint).	First 3 pints plus 20% of approved amount for additional pints (after $100 deductible).****

    * You pay the $100 Part B deductible only once each year.
   ** Federal law limits charges for physician services (see page 20)
  *** Part B pays for home health care only if you do not have Part A of Medicare.
 **** To the extent any of the three pints of blood are paid for or replaced under one part of Medicare during the calendar year, they do not have to be paid for or replaced under the other part.

1997 Part B monthly premium: $43.80 (premium may be higher if you enroll late).

This chart shows the features of the standard plans.

Standard Medigap Plans

	A	B	C	D	E	F	G	H	I	J
Basic Benefits	✓	✓	✓	✓	✓	✓	✓	✓	✓	✓
Skilled Nursing Coinsurance			✓	✓	✓	✓	✓	✓	✓	✓
Part A Deductible		✓	✓	✓	✓	✓	✓	✓	✓	✓
Part B Deductible			✓			✓				✓
Part B: Percent of Excess Actual Charge over Allowable Charge						100% ✓	80% ✓		100% ✓	100% ✓
Foreign Travel			✓	✓	✓	✓	✓	✓	✓	✓
At-Home Recovery				✓		✓			✓	✓
Basic Drugs ($1,250 limit)								✓	✓	
Extended Drugs ($3,000 limit)										✓
Preventive Care					✓					✓

Note: There are also two high-deductible ($1,500 out-of-pocket expenses) plans based on plans F and J.

8

The Politics of Medicare Reform in the 1990s
Budget Struggles, National Health Reform, and Shifting Conflicts

INTRODUCTION: THE CHANGING CONTEXT OF MEDICARE'S POLITICS IN THE 1990s

Medicare at the opening of the decade was not among the major preoccupations of American national politics. In 1991, only 3 percent of Americans polled ranked health care and/or Medicare as the most important issue facing the country (Gallup Poll, 1991, 197).[1] By the 1992 presidential campaign, however, widespread attention to Medicare returned as two distinct issues of American medical policy came into brief but intense conflict. First, there was the targeting of Medicare expenditures, which federal officials regularly forecasted to rise over the 1990s, as a way to reduce the federal budget deficit. That issue momentarily heated up the debate between the Bush and Clinton campaigns when Budget Director Richard Darman claimed in July 1992 that Medicare outlays would have to be drastically reduced if the budget deficit were to be substantially lowered. The other set of political issues involved the emergent politics of universal health insurance in the early 1990s—both the realization that an extraordinary consensus had emerged about the need for far-reaching change and the presumption that, if elected, Clinton aimed to act on that consensus.

In fact, Medicare and the medical concerns of the elderly receded into the background as the battle over the Clinton health plan dominated American politics during 1993–94. It was only in mid-1995, when the Medicare trustees forecasted the program's trust fund "insolvency" by 2002, that broad public attention was drawn once again to Medicare. Despite this attention the program continued until 1997 with few dramatic shifts in its administration, financing, or benefits. What followed in the summer of 1997, however, was major change. There were legislative adjustments in Medicare's financial structure, alteration of the terms of its payments to various health plans, and an experiment with medical savings accounts—all with important consequences for Medicare's own administration. This was not a well-thought out, considered reform of a popular program requiring adjustment. What happened in 1997 was, like the original enactment in 1965, a rather pressured, highly uncertain set of policies, adaptations to a transformed political environment (Oberlander, 1997).[2]

The context for the 1997 Medicare changes reflected two long-term forces at work in American politics. One element was the wearing down of the faith in government—and ameliorative social programs—that had been central to Medicare's birth in the heyday of the Great Society. The second was a form of fiscal politics that emphasized the consequences of the aging of the baby boomers, particularly the budgetary strain they would put on both Medicare and Social Security in the years ahead. Building on the deficit politics of the 1980s, the self-styled advocates of generational equity—figures like Wall Street financier Peter Peterson and senators Durenberger, Rudman, and Tsongas—helped disseminate the view that without major change Medicare and Social Security would become unaffordable (Marmor, Mashaw, and Harvey, 1990, 5). This presumption of great fiscal stress in the future would shape the politics of Medicare adjustment in 1997, precisely when American short-term budget circumstances had improved beyond anyone's expectations at the beginning of the decade.[3] This would not be the first, or the last time, that distorted argument—and surprise—would mark Medicare's policymaking. Nor would it be the only time that the perception of Medicare lagged behind its reality.

MEDICARE AND THE 1992 ELECTIONS: THE REAWAKENING OF CONCERNS

During the 1992 presidential campaign the Bush administration proposed a "cap" on Medicare and Medicaid in order to reduce forecasted federal health spending between 1993 and 1997 by some $260 billion. Such a policy, charged candidate Clinton, would eviscerate Medicare, let alone Medicaid. Economists advising the Clinton campaign issued dire warnings: enforcing such caps alone, absent more far-reaching healthcare reforms, would destroy Medicaid, increase cost-shifting from Medicare to employment-based insurance, and lead to the loss of millions of jobs (Thorpe, 1992).

The immediate result was a firestorm of criticism of such proposed "draconian" cuts. Although the Bush campaign claimed these criticisms were nothing but the familiar scare tactics of the Democrats, the fears about spending caps had some justification. To get Medicare savings of $145 billion between 1993 and 1997, the Bush administration's Darman proposed what seemed like impossible burdens on the elderly, hospitals, and some physicians.

A quick review makes plain why the Darman "plan" excited such outrage. To save nearly $64 billion in Medicare's physician insurance program, the proposal called for increases in the premiums and copayments for which the elderly were financially responsible. Coupled with increases in private insurance premiums for supplementary Medicare policies (Medigap), such changes, the Congressional Budget Office estimated, would have increased the elderly's spending on health care from 7 percent of their incomes to nearly 12 percent by 1997. Other proposed spending cuts under Part B ($14 billion over 5 years) presumed substantial reductions in payments to physicians (Thorpe, 1992).

That, of course, was only half the picture. The other savings—estimated at $69 billion—were to come from Medicare's hospital insurance program, Part A. In 1992, Medicare paid almost 90 percent of "reported" hospital costs (ProPac, 1992). The Darman scheme proposed to cut the rate of reimbursement to hospitals, down to roughly 72 percent of their reported costs by 1997. On the basis of past experience, hospitals were expected to shift much of those reductions to other payers. Thus, spending cuts in Medicare alone would likely have entailed higher out-of-pocket medical costs for the elderly (cost-shifting backwards), increased burdens on employers (cost-shifting sideways), and decreased revenues or higher fees for physicians (cost-shifting forward) (Moon, 1996, 7). Such shifts risked enraging those constituencies and complicating any reasonable reform of the way medical care *in general* would be organized, delivered, and financed in the future.

In the face of such criticism, President Bush tried to distance himself from the flare-up by calling his budget director's Medicare proposal merely one "option." With that campaign retreat, the Medicare program faded from public view during the remainder of the 1992 presidential race. Although Medicare faded as a campaign issue, the broader topic of medical care reform and national health insurance continued to play a major role in coloring the political climate. The general topic had, in fact, come onto the political radar screen before the 1992 campaign had assumed center stage. The real precipitant was the November 1991 election in Pennsylvania of the largely unknown Democrat Harris Wofford to fill the senatorial seat opened by the unexpected death of Republican senator John Heinz. In an instant, Wofford's upset victory over former attorney general Richard Thornburgh, widely attributed to Wofford's advocacy of universal health insurance, turned the attention of the nation's political commentators to the troubled state of American medicine. The nation's reporters—and many of its politicians—discovered that a broad social consensus had actually emerged over the 1980s that American medical care, particularly its financing and insurance coverage, needed a major overhaul (Hacker, 1997).

A NEGATIVE CONSENSUS ON HEALTH REFORM

Had George Bush won a second term as president, deficit politics and Medicare would no doubt have collided head-on. The campaign flurry of excited criticism from Democrats generally and the aging lobbies particularly would have made that all but certain. But President Clinton faced different problems in acting on the bold campaign promises he had made to reform American medical care "comprehensively." It was no longer disputed that the American system of medical care—enormously expensive by comparative standards while leaving roughly one of six Americans without insurance coverage—required substantial reform. The critical unanimity on this point bridged almost all the usual political cleavages—between old and young, Democrats and Republicans, management and labor, the well-paid and the low-paid. The U.S. spent more and felt worse than all its economic competitors. What's more, nine out of ten Americans told pollsters in the early 1990s that American medical care required very substantial change, a consensus that was also reflected in polls of Fortune 500 executives (Marmor, 1997b). This was the encouraging news for medical care reformers, whether in Congress, among interest groups, or in what would become the Clinton administration.

The bad news for reformers was, as had been the case in earlier decades, a bitter truth. A consensus on the seriousness of American medical care problems did not signify agreement on the shape, magnitude, or priority of those problems. Nor did a negative consensus bring with it agreement on remedies, as was amply demonstrated by the battle over Medicare's enactment in the 1960s. Policymakers and politicians are often surprised to discover that an overwhelming public acceptance of the need to address a given problem does not guarantee any consensus on what the best solution is to that problem. Public acceptance is merely a precondition—a crucial one, to be sure. But public acknowledgment of a problem does not ensure that an agreement can be reached on a policy resolution. In fact, the more complex the problem, like making medical care accessible to and affordable for all Americans, the less likely that such an agreement can be forged, despite widespread agreement that the situation needs fixing. In short, no one can predict the emergence of workable reform legislation from widespread acceptance of problems meriting attention. That understanding, however, was not fully apparent to the enthusiasts President Clinton brought to the White House in January 1993 (Marmor, 1993; Hacker, 1997).

There was also a serious political danger—one involving Medicare directly—that lurked just beneath the surface of the discussion of overarching, national health reform. Any comprehensive reform proposal submitted by the administration would have to gauge very carefully its potential impact on Medicare recipients. That much was apparent from the politically devastating conflict that had marked the catastrophic health insurance struggle of 1988–89 (Himelfarb, 1997). Any tampering with Medicare—even constructive tampering—risked reawakening not only further generational conflict, but the opposition of a powerfully organized constituency: America's senior citizens. As Martin Corry, the director of federal affairs for the American Association of Retired People, warned at the time, "Whenever you talk about changes in Medicare, it makes people nervous" (*New York Times*, May 1993). What's more, the very effectiveness of the 1992 attack on the Darman proposals, an attack led by the Clinton campaign, only reinforced the Clinton administration's sensitivity to the risks of changing Medicare.

There was no question that Medicare needed some adjustment, as do all programs over time. But it became a subject of scrutiny following Clinton's election not because of a public perception that Medicare needed modification, but because of its sheer fiscal size. Within what many Americans viewed as the uncontrollable world of medical inflation, Medicare appeared a vigorous consumer of public dollars. On its historical trajectory, an unreformed Medicare was certain to make deficit reduction difficult, if not impossible. And, by 1993, deficit reduction was accepted as a first-order political objective. As president, Clinton confronted this reality directly in his first economic report to the Congress. Any effort to make good on his promise to cut the budget deficit in half by 1996 meant President Clinton had to show how Medicare outlays would be constrained. After all, the economic plan he released during the campaign had promised "savings" of billions in Medicare outlays, a sharp contrast to the Bush administration's fearful forecasts that uncapped Medicare expenditures would grow at 15.8 percent annually. Those deficit savings had to come from either reductions in what Medicare paid out or increased Medicare taxes, or both. But how could the Clinton administration get Medicare's outlays under control without the full fright (and fight) associated with the 1992 suggestion to cap Medicare expenditures we have already noted?

The prospects for bringing Medicare expenditures under control were, in fact, considerably better than most Americans—and most members of Congress—realized at that time. During its first two decades, Medicare's costs had undeniably grown rapidly, rising from 9.2 percent of national health expenditures in 1967 to 16.7 percent in 1984 (see Figure 8.1). The program reimbursed hospitals their "reasonable costs," and paid physicians their "reasonable and customary fees." But the financial results were, as Chapter 7 revealed, neither reasonable nor customary. Medicare *appeared* to be a program whose costs were always rising faster than the nation's income.

The Congressional Budget Office then reinforced this dire view of Medicare's finances by projecting that the program's outlays would increase by approximately 11 percent *every* year from 1993 to 1997. But this pessimistic picture of Medicare's future was actually at odds with the facts. Between 1980 and 1991 the rate of increase in Medicare outlays had fallen sharply, from an average annual rate of just over 16 percent between 1980 and 1985 to an average of 8.2 percent between 1986 and 1991. Thus in fact the rate of increase in the late 1980s was well below the 11 percent rate used in the projections of either the Bush administration in 1990 or the CBO in 1992 (see Figure 8.2).

What made Medicare's performance even more striking was this: the program had also controlled its outlays more tightly than did private health insurers during the period 1983–93 (see Figure 7.5; Moon and Zuckerman, 1995; Reinhardt, 1997). And if stronger federal action were to be implemented, the rate of increase in Medicare expenditures could, it seemed, be brought down to a level approaching that of general inflation, not two or three times that figure. However, as is often the case with American public policy, perception lagged behind reality. Attention to forecasts of dramatic growth in Medicare expenditures was to increase—because of heightened interest in the reduction of the federal budget—at the end of a decade in which the growth in Medicare's outlays had slowed considerably.

Even had Medicare expenditures increased less than expected, the potential impact of those federal outlays on Clinton's plan for universal health coverage remained substantial. Successful efforts by the Clinton administration to tighten controls on Medicare costs[4] would still have risked exacerbating the worrisome trend in health finance that took place during the 1980s: the shifting of Medicare expenses from public accounts to other payers, including private insurance companies and patients. That is, unless cost restraints were imposed throughout the medical economy—whether enforced through price and volume con-

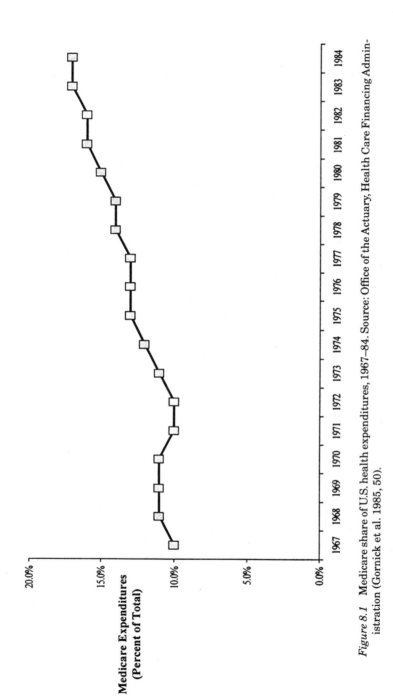

Figure 8.1 Medicare share of U.S. health expenditures, 1967–84. Source: Office of the Actuary, Health Care Financing Administration (Gornick et al. 1985, 50).

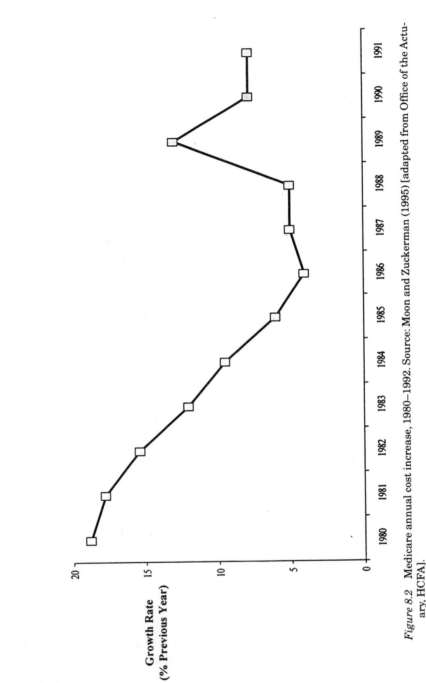

Figure 8.2 Medicare annual cost increase, 1980–1992. Source: Moon and Zuckerman (1995) [adapted from Office of the Actuary, HCFA].

trols, as in Medicare, or through the "managed competition" plan that Clinton subsequently proposed—financial controls on Medicare alone would *shift* as well as restrain medical costs. That, in turn, would have risked introducing another element into the fray: the generational conflict between older Americans who felt entitled to Medicare's benefits and those younger Americans who felt they were bearing an increased and unfair burden in order to make Medicare affordable to its present beneficiaries. The potential for this conflict was serious. Critics could have been expected to seize on the image of "greedy geezers" as a plausible explanation for the nation's budget and other woes. (Though this view has never attracted majority support, it has been widely advertised and, in its less angry form, commands respectful attention.)

Underlying this charge of unaffordability is a very different view of the proper role of government in social welfare policy. The advocates for reducing America's programs for the elderly, such as the Americans for Generational Equity (1990) and the Concord Coalition (1992), espouse a more limited role for public programs in general—something closer to the Poor Law tradition as opposed to the social insurance ideology that has largely dominated American social policy since the depression. And it is not surprising that the enthusiasts for deficit reduction turned their sights on Medicare and Social Security in the 1980s and 1990s. The systematic reduction of federal social welfare efforts, especially those for children and youth in the Reagan/Bush era, left little else but the elderly programs to turn to for fiscal savings.

Of course, these two conceptions parallel almost exactly the welfare and social security approaches distinguished in Chapter 2, and the charity and middle-class programs analyzed in Chapter 5. In this respect, there was little new about the criticism of social insurance except the fiscal fears and the occasional portrait of the elderly as excessively demanding. Throughout the 1980s and 1990s, political and fiscal conservatives were able to rally attention and concern for their frightening budgetary portrait of the present and the future. The current young, they repeatedly insisted, would be deprived of economic opportunities and future well-being because of the excessive allocation of resources to the old (Quadagno, 1989).

This claim of generational inequity proved intermittently divisive in the social policy politics in these decades. Indeed, the pressure group that most prominently emerged—Americans for Generational Equity—found its fortunes waxing and waning (Americans for Generational Equity, 1990). Much of their forecasting was unjustified hyperbole and, beyond that, there was no documented evidence at all that the American public was hostile to the country's older citizens or to Medicare and Social Security (Jacobs, Shapiro, and Schulman, 1993). Yet, the regular dissemination of the assertion that the United States could not afford its level of generosity to the elderly without harming future generations affected the context in which Medicare came to be understood. The premise of budgetary unaffordability made budget restraint seem a prudent, not a punishing proposal. The conventions of American public debate are such that repeated and exaggerated claims of crises are seldom exposed or corrected. This made it almost certain that the affordability of America's programs for the elderly would continue to be a source of tension in any future discussions of Medicare. As the baby boomers approach retirement in the second decade of the twenty-first century, the appeals to such tensions are certain to become even more intense.

Like the periodic references to "crisis" whenever Medicare's trust fund comes within seven years of what the accountants call "insolvency" (Oberlander, 1995), the appeals to generational equity have become covert attacks on social insurance programs. When such programs are broadly popular—as with Medicare and Social Security—the most promising way to try to undercut support has been to claim either unfairness or unaffordability. While Medicare remained untouched politically during the first half of the 1990s, this legacy of questioning Medicare's fairness and fiscal affordability would have a major effect on its politics and structure in the later half of the decade.

There were in principle more straightforward ways to address Medicare's fiscal problems that would have avoided inflaming the generational equity issue while nevertheless controlling the program's expenditures and minimizing cost-shifting. The obvious option would have been to enact universal health insurance, fold Medicare into it, and impose controls on payments to providers (an approach that had already proved so successful within Medicare in the 1980s). For such a reform to have been successful, there would have had to be budget setting nationwide or statewide limits on total medical expenditures, and the elderly would have needed to be provided at least the same level of benefits under the new regime as they had had under Medicare.

A working model of such a system was Canada's national health insurance, where provincial governments act as single insurers. There was much to say in favor of Canada's approach. With universal coverage for its citizens and freedom of choice in selecting primary-care physicians, the Canadian system was considerably less expensive than that of the United States. (In 1996, Canada spent about 9.5 percent of its national income on medical care; the U.S. figure for that year was approximately 14 percent.) A survey of ten industrialized nations found that Canadians were the most satisfied with their healthcare system, Americans the least (Blendon et al., 1990). One study published in the mid-1980s plausibly suggested that the United States could have saved upwards of $65 billion per year in administrative costs alone by cutting out the 1500 private insurers and going to a single government insurer in each state—enough savings to cover, without imposing any additional cost controls, the more than 30 million Americans who were then uninsured (Himmelstein and Woolhandler, 1986).

No matter what the potential advantages of Canada's national health insurance, however, and no matter how seriously study groups may once have considered it, President Clinton regarded the idea as politically infeasible (Marmor and Hamburger, 1993). Indeed, a year before his election in November 1992, candidate Clinton had firmly rejected the Canadian model. He feared that both Republicans and the medical establishment would never weary of crying "socialized medicine," the well-worn phrase these same constituencies had used before in opposing Medicare (Marmor, Hamburger, and Meacham, 1994). As a New Democrat who distanced himself from the New Deal and Great Society programs, candidate Clinton was especially anxious to avoid any socialist label. What's more, this advertised position (New Democrat) made increased taxes and direct government administration of health insurance appear untenable.

The Clinton administration's strategy was, instead, to reach universal coverage by a combination of indirect steps and at the same time to set in place the elements of overall cost control (Hacker, 1997). Rejecting a single-payer system for all Americans and favoring one of managed competition among different health plans, the Clinton administration proposed requiring employers to offer health insurance, with a backup public program for the unemployed. The plan suggested folding Medicaid into state corporations chartered to purchase health insurance. But, mindful of the political clout of the elderly and the public outcry against Medicare cuts during the 1992 campaign, Clinton's plan proposed leaving the Medicare program more or less as it was. To be sure, there was a proposed option for Medicare beneficiaries to join non-Medicare health alliances and thereby reap the presumed rewards of managed competition. Medicare beneficiaries who chose to move to the new health alliances would not be guaranteed to receive any additional benefits or services (Hacker, 1997). As in the early 1970s, Medicare was once again subordinated to national health reform. This time, however, the suppression was more out of fear of antagonizing Medicare constituents than out of optimism of the reformers.

President Clinton hoped to produce by the end of his first term a coherent amalgam of the fragmented pieces euphemistically called the "American medical care system." Yet this approach quelled neither the concerns of the elderly nor the fiscal anxieties of critics. The elderly did not believe that the proposals adequately protected their interests. Nor did the critics believe that this approach addressed the problem of bringing further necessary controls on Medicare expenditures.

In an attempt to gain the support of the elderly for its major reform proposal, the administration did, in fact, propose adding some additional Medicare benefits: coverage for prescription drugs, as well as long-term care for the severely disabled. The issue of long-term care was otherwise not addressed. Not surprisingly, these modest carrots failed to win the support of AARP and other groups speaking for the elderly. Testifying before Congress and making national news in the process, Judith Brown, the director of AARP, emphasized the worry that "individuals who decided to join the Medicare program would be subject to higher cost-sharing, no cap on out-of-pocket costs and less generous low-income protections—in short, worse coverage than that available through regional alliances." Ms. Brown summarized AARP's response with language clearly suggesting that the Clinton administration had failed to rally support among the elderly's most prominent pressure group: "We are deeply disappointed that the President's plan would not provide the same coverage for Medicare beneficiaries as it would for younger populations" (House Committee on Ways and Means, 1993). Yet Brown also warned that alliances might ill-serve the elderly: "Currently, there is a system in place that is generally responsive to the special vulnerability of the Medicare population. . . . For those who are most physically dependent on the system, we believe that it is prudent to preserve a program with a good track record, at least until the new system has proven successful." Ironically, the AARP withheld support both because the proposals might result in Medicare beneficiaries who chose to join health alliances receiving *worse* benefits than under traditional Medicare, and because the health alliances held out the possibility of providing *better* benefits than Medicare.

The Clinton administration's reform plan provided no clear proposals for bringing Medicare expenditures under tighter control. This omission guaranteed that Medicare would, at some future point, once again come under political attack, especially considering its substantial impact on the federal budget. By 1995, Medicare constituted 10.5 percent of the federal budget, compared to 3.5 percent in 1970 (Moon, 1996, 2).

In the end, of course, the Clinton administration's effort to enact "comprehensive" medical care reform ended in humiliating defeat. The plan's slow death in September 1994 prompted a furious and continuing round of blaming, exculpatory rhetoric, and scholarly reconstruction (including Fallows, 1995; Hacker, 1997; Marmor and Mashaw, 1996; Steinmo and Watts, 1995; White, 1995; Yankelovich, 1995). It is

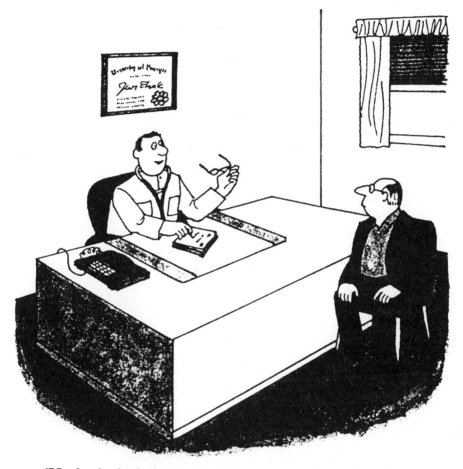

"You're in luck, in a way. Now is the time to be sick—
while Medicare still has some money."

worth noting, though, that even if the Clinton reform plan had succeeded, it would have failed to confront the most crucial problems Medicare faced. The fears and concerns of the elderly would have remained largely unaddressed. Medicare expenditures would have remained under no new restraints. The problem of cost-shifting may very well have continued to undermine efforts to control medical care expenditures fairly. The nation's capacity to afford the costs of both Medicare and the rest of American medicine would have been severely tested, as would the associated efforts to reduce the federal deficit (Marmor, 1993). Acting within the constraints of what it regarded as politically feasible, the Clinton administration opted for a reform plan comprised of managed competition and regional alliances, leaving Medicare largely alone.

THE 1995 TRUSTEES' REPORT AND CLAIMS OF INSOLVENCY

The discussion of Medicare and its problems practically disappeared from the national public agenda during the Clinton health reform struggle. But that did not remain so for very long. Media attention returned to Medicare just as soon as the 1995 report of the trustees forecast fiscal trouble. The hospital insurance trust fund, the trustees projected, would be insolvent (or bankrupt) by 2002 if revenues and outlays behaved as currently estimated. In the language of the actuaries, that would take place when reserves would no longer be sufficient to pay the program's promised benefits.

The talk of Medicare's bankruptcy once again became commonplace, the intermingling of the vocabularies of trust funds, solvency, and fiscal prudence that has been such a central (and ambiguous) feature of social insurance politics in America since the New Deal. Clarifying the language is a precondition to understanding the fiscal politics of a program like Medicare.

In the first place, one should remember that no precise analog to private bankruptcy exists in public programs like Medicare. The program's hospital "trust fund," for example, refers to an accounting term, a conventional way to describe earmarked revenue and spending. The very notion of a public trust fund emphasized the trust that the earmarked financing was meant to symbolize. So, for instance, the Medicare reformers had taken for granted that wage-related taxes paid by workers would fully (and legitimately) finance hospital benefits for retired workers. Since 1936, federal agencies had used the language of trust and the reality of wage-related taxes as funding sources to underscore the solidity of commitment to finance promised benefits in social insurance programs. Other agencies of government came to use this same device to describe specially favored (and protected) objects of governmental support (Patashnik, 2000). By the late twentieth century, Americans had grown so used to such accounting conventions that the differences in private and public financing had become indistinct.

In private firms or households, a trust fund without funds is literally insolvent, unable to finance any activity. Trusts cannot tax and their other options are highly constrained. It makes sense to think of trustees making sure the projected income from the trust fund's investments are financially realistic; there is no place else to turn if the invested capital is lost or the income sharply reduced. Congress, on the other hand, has a radically different relation to the financing and spending decisions affecting trust fund programs like Medicare. It can, for example, change the hospital tax rate for Medicare and immediately eliminate any shortfall, if it has the political will to do so. Likewise, the Congress can alter the benefits and reimbursement provisions of the program's hospital or medical coverage. Or it can do some of both, as it has in different proportions over Medicare's operational history since 1966. Channeling the financial consequences of these decisions through a trust fund does not change the real political economy of Medicare. In short, the trust associated with the fund is a psychologically important, but fiscally neutral element in the goods and services Medicare finances. A particular Congress (or administration) may, of course, fail to fulfill its promise and in that sense violate popular trust. But that is because it lacks the political will or ability to tax more or spend less, or because the country itself is unable to do either because of political turmoil. It is not because the trust funds have simply run low. Thinking that the trust fund is the crucial fiscal variable is analogous to thinking that a thermometer's reading constitutes a heat wave or a freeze.[5] Fiscal strain and political stress—that language accurately describes Medicare's budget circumstances in the mid-1990s and after. As we will explore further, there is a recurrent pattern to periods of crisis talk in Medicare.

The oddity of worrying about a Medicare bankruptcy is also apparent when one considers the different political responses to the funding shortfalls for Medicare's hospitalization coverage, on the one hand, and to the shortfalls for its coverage for physician services, on the other. Hospitalization insurance alone, as Part I of this volume emphasized, was the original focus of those who drafted the initial Medicare legislation. And it was this hospital coverage that payroll taxes paid throughout workers' lives would finance. These taxes were earmarked for Medicare's Part A trust fund, which in turn is the formal source of financing for the hospital expenses of the program's beneficiaries. Designed along the same social-insurance principles as Social Security pensions, the goal was to provide universal hospital coverage as an earned benefit, rather than as a charity payment, to all those who had contributed during their working lives.

As explained in Chapter 5, only a surprising last-minute move by Wilbur Mills added coverage for physician services in 1965 to the Medicare bill as Part B. But unlike hospital coverage, physician expenses were to be financed by premium payments from current beneficiaries and by general federal tax revenues. Because general tax revenues can only run *short*—but not *out*—projected shortfalls in paying for physician services have simply been covered by additional general revenues, by increased premiums, or by cutbacks in expenditures. As a consequence, there have never been Medicare Part B crises of the form associated with Part A. It is only the projected shortfalls in the hospital trust fund that have triggered the recurrent crises over Medicare and the use of bankruptcy language. Perversely, the same social-insurance financing of hospital services that was so critical to gaining political support for Medicare in the first place has—through its artifact, the trust fund—become one of its greatest political vulnerabilities and the nominal foundation to support the attacks of the program's harshest critics (Oberlander, 1995). The experience with the trust fund demonstrates how important the funding mechanisms can be for the politics of a program. To that extent, the use of a trust fund is more than an accounting term of art. It has very real political implications and consequences.

These attacks on Medicare have arisen at predictable points in Medicare's history. As Jon Oberlander has established, the three Medicare "crises"—in 1969, 1983, and 1995—all came at the point that Medicare's actuaries projected the trust fund's exhaustion within *seven* years (see Figure 8.3). With the program appearing vulnerable according to official reports, and with projected financial shortfalls sufficiently tangible to engage public attention, critics as well as supporters have seized upon the metaphor of "insolvency" to make program changes more palatable. The predicted troubles of the trust fund provide a seemingly prudent rationale for transforming the program itself (Oberlander, 1995). And it was just such an attack that was triggered by the 1995 trustees' report.

FROM LEGISLATIVE IMPASSE 1995–96 TO MEDICARE "REFORM" IN 1997

Republicans, led by then Speaker of the House Newt Gingrich, bolstered by their victories in the 1994 congressional elections, and united

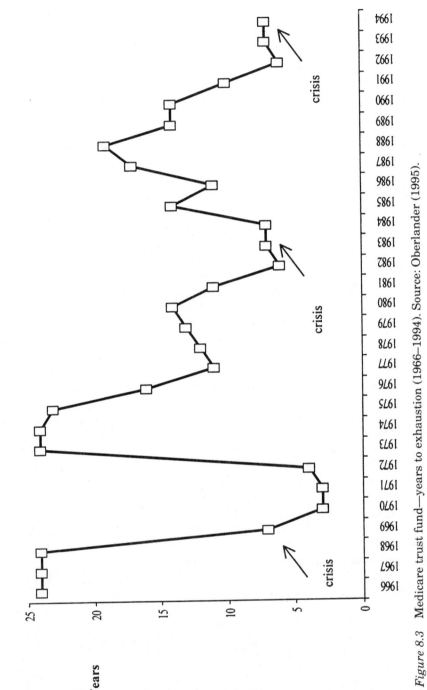

Figure 8.3 Medicare trust fund—years to exhaustion (1966–1994). Source: Oberlander (1995).

by their Contract with America's fierce attack on the American welfare state, immediately seized upon the trustees' forecast of fiscal trouble by 2002.[6] For them it signaled yet another looming Medicare crisis and justified a radical and immediate cutback in program expenditures. The Republicans labeled their proposal the "Medicare Preservation Act of 1995" and argued that to "preserve, protect, and strengthen" Medicare required reductions of $270 billion in projected spending over the next seven years (a figure that was suspiciously close to the $245 billion in tax cuts the Republicans also proposed, mostly for the affluent). Democrats charged in response that Republican preservation meant Medicare's destruction. Representative Charles Rangel of New York went so far as to say that the Republican proposal put American "grandmothers . . . in jeopardy" (*Chicago Tribune,* September 22, 1995). This acrimonious debate left most citizens perplexed—as much by its partisan fury as by its largely incomprehensible budgetary jargon. The nation's elderly and disabled were understandably worried.

President Clinton, though avoiding rhetoric that strident, nonetheless was sharply critical of the Republicans' proposed cutbacks in Medicare expenditures. He adamantly defended America's commitment to take care of its elderly citizens and presented his own plan to bring Medicare expenditures under control. But since President Clinton proposed reductions of $128 billion in projected outlays—or approximately half that of the Republican proposal—his plan had no realistic chance of enactment by the Republican-controlled Congress of 1995. An impasse developed, with Republican charges of demagoguery against the Democrats and Democratic charges of Republican heartlessness. During this impasse the public opinion tables turned. It was President Clinton and the Democrats who emerged as the defenders of Medicare, as the polls documented (Rushefsky and Patel, 1998, 208–9, 237–38). House Speaker Gingrich, on the other hand, came out of the tangle rather tarnished, in part through his own zealousness in attacking American social welfare programs in general. By early 1996, the Contract with America had lost much of its attraction, and the Republican majority lost most of its political momentum (Hacker, 1997). Calls of crisis were renewed when it became apparent that Medicare's trust fund would be "empty" even sooner than the 2002 date trustees had projected in their 1995 report (*Washington Post,* 1996). Despite that fear-mongering, the Republicans were still unable to overcome the Democrats' opposition to a radical overhaul on Medicare. The result of this continuing partisan conflict was a bitterly divided Congress and legislative inertia on Medicare as the presidential election approached in the summer of 1996.

In their enthusiasm for reform, the Republicans had been defeated by some of the same elements that had previously doomed President

Clinton's effort to enact universal health insurance. Despite a negative consensus that Medicare needed fiscal adjustment, Republicans failed to establish a positive consensus on what needed to be done. The reasons for this failure—both with Medicare and other Republican reform efforts—were clear to some observers. Republicans made a number of mistaken and costly assumptions that led to the loss of the political advantage they had gained in the 1994 elections. They presumed to govern the country from Congress, taking for granted that President Clinton would simply surrender politically and let them have their way. Furthermore, Republican leaders assumed their electoral mandate from 1994 was so strong that they could substantially cut back even such popular programs as Medicare. A final Republican mistake was refusing to bargain politically with the Democrats to achieve an agreement on budget restraint. As a consequence, rather than obtaining very significant budgetary reductions and dividing Democrats in Congress over the wisdom of political accommodation with their opponents, the Republicans held their ground, their poll ratings collapsed, and President Clinton emerged a rehabilitated leader (Dionne, 1996).

If we examine the legislative impasse over Medicare from 1995 to 1996, we see that much more was at stake than whether Democrats and Republicans would reach a reasonable compromise on the Medicare budget. The battle was not just over Medicare, but over the future structure of the American welfare state. Republican leaders believed the time was ripe for a challenge to the social-insurance principles underlying both Medicare and Social Security.[7] They controlled both houses of Congress for the first time in 40 years and Medicare obviously needed some adjustments, both short- and long-term. At the same time, there was a perception among Washington elites of widespread public support for controlling government spending to contain the federal deficit. Moreover, the prospective retirement of the baby boomers beginning in 2010 figured prominently in the picture of an American government facing a tidal wave of expenses from programs directed at the growing number of elderly citizens.[8]

The rhetoric of generational equity was part of this apocalyptic conception of the future. It enabled some welfare state critics to defend demands for budgetary restrictions without exposing their ideological opposition to popular programs like Medicare. In 1995 and 1996, however, the fiscal fear tactics used to justify major Medicare program changes backfired. The debate in that period—with the Republicans frequently described as extremist and dangerous to senior citizens—contributed enormously to the president's improved reputation and his reelection in 1996 (Rushefsky and Patel, 1998). That makes all the more puzzling why, within a year, the Congress and the president would agree on not only the most far-reaching Medicare policy changes since its enactment, but reforms strikingly similar to what the Republicans had unsuccessfully demanded in 1995 (Oberlander, 1999).

THE MEDICARE REFORMS OF 1997: UNDERSTANDING THE POLITICS OF BALANCING BUDGETS

In August 1997 the Clinton administration and the Republican-controlled Congress agreed to a sweeping package of reforms in Medicare as part of the 1997 Balanced Budget Act. Reforms here means substantial changes in policy (reform), not necessarily improvement, though many celebrated the legislation at the time as an example of bipartisan cooperation (Etheredge, 1997). Indeed, with the exception of a few outspoken critics, such as Democratic Congressman Stark of California, both political parties endorsed the changes, as did the American Medical Association and the American Association of Retired Persons (Oberlander, 1999). How did it happen that the partisan acrimony of the 1995–96 battles gave way to bipartisan celebration of the very program changes that provoked the earlier fury? Reviewing the changes alone—or their merits— reveals what happened, but not why.

The Medicare provisions of the Balanced Budget Act, according to one expert observer, evolved out of two years of political battle between President Clinton and the Congress over the terms of any budget-balancing proposal. Medicare was at the center of that contest, with

> one of the key issues . . . whether Medicare could and should be made more like the private sector in which, supposedly, savings were being realized while employees were being given a choice among types of coverage. The alternative was to save money in ways that reflected experience with Medicare itself: through some mix of tightening of the PPS [hospital] and MVPS [physician payment] systems, correction of the problems with the Medicare Risk program, and perhaps higher charges to beneficiaries. The answer was, both! The Balanced Budget Act saved money in the traditional way, while including measures to make Medicare more like the private sector insurance world (White, 1998, p. 29). (Oberlander, 1999)

The mix of traditional and nontraditional forms of cost control and program reform was projected to save substantial federal funds over time. What was not anticipated was the reluctance of Medicare beneficiaries to take up the new options, which meant in turn that traditional cost control would dominate the implementation of the 1997 changes.[9]

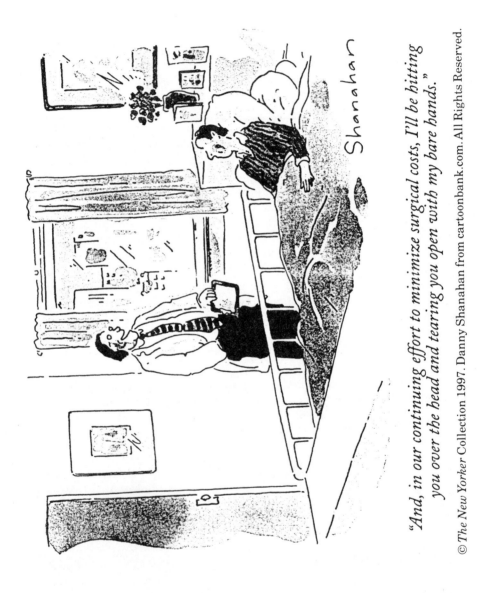

"And, in our continuing effort to minimize surgical costs, I'll be hitting you over the head and tearing you open with my bare hands."

The role of Medicare reform in the balancing of the federal budget, as the figure illustrates, actually arose primarily from reduced growth in the fee-for-service program (Moon, 1996, 6).

As a result, understanding the 1997 changes requires a sharp distinction between short term effects and policy changes aimed to transform the program over the longer run. The 1997 legislation undoubtedly included a variety of quite new elements. While discussing the policy changes in detail is beyond the scope of this chapter, it is important to note the innovations directed toward making Medicare resemble more closely the insurance terms most Americans faced by 1997. For example, the budget act proposed opening up Medicare more widely than ever before to private health insurance companies. The share of beneficiaries expected to leave the public Medicare program for private plans—through the Medicare + Choice option—was substantial.[10] Advocates claimed this change would benefit Medicare's fiscal position; the program, they argued, could take advantage of managed care's supposed virtues so as to control Medicare's spending.[11] But scant attention in 1997 was paid to the substantial difficulties that opening Medicare up to private insurance companies might impose. Nor was there much commentary about the probability that America's older citizens would or would not embrace these new options. Instead, what followed was largely a legislative celebration of the possible benefits of having Medicare resemble the private provision of care, and less a realistic analysis of how Medicare might fit into contemporary medical patterns in the private sector. In the rush to close a budget deal, Medicare policy changed radically. The question, mostly unasked at the time, was whether and how Medicare would deal with the problems facing privately insured Americans.

One such identified problem, for instance, was risk selection (sometimes known as cream skimming). This is the process by which insurers try to enroll (or keep) healthier, cheaper patients and to avoid (or shed) sicker, more expensive patients. This problem had faced Medicare before 1997. Indeed, the earlier HMO contracts had proven lucrative to capitated plans precisely because Medicare beneficiaries healthier than average brought with them capitation payments that assumed a near random selection of beneficiaries (Oberlander, 1999).

Past risk selection in Medicare threatened to get worse under the terms of the 1997 legislation. More private insurers eagerly sought an expansion of their share of the reformed Medicare market. But which part of the market did they want? Medicare costs, after all, are highly concentrated. In 1996, for example, the most expensive 10 percent of program beneficiaries averaged $37,000 in medical expenditures and accounted for 75.5 percent of all program costs (Moon, 1996, 2). In the new Medicare market, private insurers could be expected to compete aggressively to avoid enrolling such costly patients, leaving them for the public Medicare program. The resulting dynamic appeared all too predictable. The costs of public Medicare would rise because its patient pool would be sicker and thus more expensive over time. Critics would point to the rise as evidence of government ineptitude, however inaccurate that might be. Meanwhile, with the Medicare insurance pool fragmented in countless directions, the federal government would in effect pay bonuses to private plans that avoid sick patients (Oberlander, 1999).

These projected costs of risk selection were so significant that the Congressional Budget Office predicted Medicare would actually lose money under several of the new health plans (Congressional Budget Office, 1997). In particular, Medical Savings Accounts and provider-sponsored organizations were expected by most analysts to attract relatively healthy beneficiaries. At least in the short run, moving Medicare toward the private market seemed to promise ending up *costing,* not saving, the program money. That was the common complaint in 1997 of those concerned about the threats presented by the innovative provisions of the Balanced Budget Acts treatment of Medicare (Marmor and Hacker, 1997).

However, neither the reform optimists nor the pessimistic critics of the 1997 legislation proved prescient. Few older Americans took up either the expanded managed care options or the new medical savings account.[12] What fiscal savings took place arose from the use of traditional cost control instruments, whether threatened or applied. Popular with some Washington elites, the Medicare innovations of 1997 did not arise from public demands. As a result a central puzzle remains in dealing with the most substantial alteration of the Medicare program in 30 years: why did the legislation pass when it did and in that form?

The rationale for reform was simple, but cannot explain either the legislation itself or its implementation. The changes in the private medical care sector that swept the nation in the 1990s—the so-called managed care revolution—provided for some advocates a model for Medicare. At the core of the reform perspective was the belief, as Jon Oberlander has written, that "Medicare should substantially increase the enrollment of [its beneficiaries] in managed care plans" (Oberlander, 1995). To do so, according to supporters, promised greater cost control, wider choices available to Medicare's beneficiaries, improved medical quality, and, most prominently, bringing Medicare in line with private sector developments (Marmor and Oberlander, 1998). None of these claims were (or are) obviously true and little of the debate addressed what many analysts knew to be exaggerated claims (Oberlander, 1999; White 1998). It is not this private sector rationale that explains the Medicare changes of 1997, but more complicated combinations of politics, policy, and circumstance.

One must look first to significant changes in the political climate surrounding Medicare. The limited public understanding of Medicare's social insurance roots and programmatic assumptions was one reason the program became vulnerable to fiscal, philosophical, and administrative attacks in the mid-1990s. To understand how a broadly supported program could shift from the status of sacred cow to endangered species requires shifting the level of analysis to broader elements in recent American politics. In particular, it means emphasizing the cumulative impact of more than two decades of questioning the affordability of the social insurance programs of the New Deal and the Great Society (Marmor, Mashaw, and Harvey, 1990). It also requires attending to how fiscal pressures—heightened by the bipartisan agreement to reach a balanced budget early in the twenty-first century—helped in the very difficult political task of making restrictions on the elderly's entitlements seem like necessary adjustments to the realities of modern American life. To this must be added increased scrutiny of Medicare in the wake of highly publicized instances of Medicare fraud in the late 1980s and into the 1990s. Attacks on the welfare state that had begun in the 1980s—and the fear the country could not continue to afford the social programs it had enacted earlier—set the stage for Medicare reform sometime, but did not determine precisely when.

The timing of major policy changes—whether in governments or large firms—is almost never a simple matter of responses to worsening problems. That is the perspective Chapter 5 identified as highly misleading, the view of a government as a rational unitary actor measuring difficulties, identifying the costs and benefits of various remedies, and selecting the best solution to the problem at hand. Thinking of the 1997 Medicare reforms this way explains neither the timing nor the content of the policy changes, let alone their operational consequences. What is required to explain the reforms is the conjunction of relevant policy ideas with both political opportunity and conventionally understood problems (Tuohy, 1999). Looked at that way, the timing and the content of the 1997 legislation are not really puzzling.

Most simply put, the ideas embedded in the 1997 reforms—both traditional and innovative—had been around throughout the 1990s. The Republican takeover of the Congress in 1994 gave the new majority a special bargaining position with the president over any big fiscal measure he strongly supported. So, when President Clinton took on a balanced budget by 2002 as his central commitment in 1997, that made a

deal with the Republicans necessary. The key condition of the deal—a
substantial reduction of Medicare's forecasted expenditures to help
balance the budget—required that the legislation's provisions satisfy
both the Clinton administration and the Republican majority. It also
meant the provisions should not precipitate a revolt among congressional Democrats. All of this, unlike the great health reform battles earlier in the decade, took place largely in private, kept out of most of the
news, with the public largely uninformed.

This understanding of the context makes sense of the most prominent 1997 results: budget savings largely through traditional Medicare
controls long acceptable to Democrats, plus a series of Medicare
changes—from medical savings accounts to the aggressive expansion of
private managed care options—ideologically appealing to Republicans.
This is essentially a story of an extended partisan battle over Medicare
since 1995 and a resulting insider deal in 1997. It explains most of the
features of what otherwise would be quite puzzling in the history of
Medicare policymaking (Peterson, 1998).

This account is unusual, but rather consistent with a number of
political science interpretations. The Republican control of the Congress was the dominant new feature of the legislative maneuvering
over the entire period 1995–97 (Oberlander, 1999; Rushefsky and Patel,
1998; Peterson, 1998; White, 1998). The framework of policy debate
changed substantially. What core programs the federal government
should continue to run became a central question, not what new items
should be added to the national agenda. Appeal to a smaller federal
government became even more rhetorically commonplace. The claim of
widespread public support for aggressive reductions of the federal
deficit was a familiar refrain. Criticism of Medicare's administration
became more common, a disillusionment fueled in part by publicity surrounding Medicare fraud. This in turn bolstered Republican claims
that the private sector and market forces could both save Medicare dollars and yet provide superior benefits. Whether managed competition
within Medicare was administratively feasible was never extensively
discussed. At the same time, the Republicans were acutely aware of
how their Medicare positions had been used against them in 1995 and
1996 and were unwilling to lead a public attack on the program's core
arrangements.

President Clinton, as noted, could not get his fiscal deal without
Republican support. Republicans, mindful of the past, would not agree
to any plan in which Democrats failed to share any blame for making
changes in Medicare. So the seeds of an insider deal were sown; neither
side had anything to gain from making the debate or the detailed bargaining public. Both sides had a lot to gain from making a deal that

allowed each to claim credit for balancing the federal budget.[13] It was that bargain, one few Americans understood, that makes sense of the 1997 changes. And, just as most Americans had no idea of how Medicare was born, few in 1997 had any understanding of how it was transformed.

MEDICARE FLIP-FLOP

A satisfactory account of what happened to Medicare between 1995 and 1999 will require (and should prompt) considerable scholarly investigation in the years to come. The main features of the story, however, are clear. The Republicans promoted vouchers for Medicare in their 1995 effort to remake American social policy, but President Clinton vetoed the bill and ran his 1996 reelection campaign in part as a defender of what later came to be called traditional Medicare. Convinced after the election that a balanced budget was a desirable legacy, Clinton made common cause with a longstanding Republican article of faith. But with balancing the budget came the need to reduce sharply Medicare's forecasted general revenue expenditures and that in turn required congressional-presidential cooperation. The price of that cooperation was acceptance of Republican reforms of Medicare along with those already favored by congressional Democrats, a development we have already sketched.

What happened then was fateful, but largely unanticipated. The 1997 Balanced Budget Act authorized a Bipartisan Commission on the Future of Medicare. While the bipartisan title implied the prospect of consensual and careful deliberation, the reality was a group of ideological opposites. The commission's leaders—Senator John Breaux (D., La.) and Congressman Bill Thomas (R., Calif.)—were both well-known critics of the growth of entitlements generally and social insurance programs like Medicare particularly. And for the most part they used the commission's work to advance their own vision of Medicare reform—the voucher plan of 1995 adjusted and relabeled as "premium support." Predictably, this met with the fierce opposition of the liberal Democrats on the commission and the whole effort came to a close in March 1999 without a formal recommendation. The stalemate ensued because the commission's ground rules required a supermajority (at least 11 of 17 members) to transmit a formal proposal to the Congress and the president, and seven of the Democrats firmly opposed the Breaux-Thomas plan. Though the commission disbanded in March, the battle over Medicare reform was hardly over. The commission chairmen introduced their proposal in the Congress in May 1999, and their bill prompted weeks of hearings and substantial media coverage. This, then, is the truncated sketch of what took place. But one does not require the full details of how this surprising story unfolded to understand its key determinants.

First, procompetitive proposals like the Breaux-Thomas plan were among the available reform options in part because of the tireless work of policy entrepreneurs inside and outside the medical care community (Oliver, 1996). Second, the Republican domination of the Congress after 1994 came to limit sharply what a Democratic president could affirmatively accomplish without bipartisan support. As long as the fight was over whether to balance the budget, Democrats could rail against Republican proposals to "cut" Medicare severely. And they did precisely that—and did so successfully—in the presidential race of 1996. But if a balanced budget bill was to be enacted, the president and the Republican majority would have to find common ground. There would have to be political credit for both parties and, in addition, the balanced budget would require substantial reductions in Medicare's projected expenditures that both parties could accept. Those budgetary reductions took place in 1997 through a combination of traditional and innovative policy adjustments in Medicare, an amalgam of what Democrats had used for cost control and what appealed to Republican market reform advocates, as we have noted.

Support grew in 1998–99 for what amounted to a policy turnaround, a transformation of Medicare into a version of Clinton's once-maligned managed competition. The reason for this is complicated. Partly it has to do with the conversion of Republican leaders to the idea of vouchers for Medicare. This began with Congressman Bill Thomas, for example, in 1995 through the prodding of the American Medical Association. The AMA, traditionally supportive of increased patient cost-sharing to control Medicare's expenditures, became convinced by mid-1995 that vouchers were the best way to cut Medicare and protect physician incomes (Castellblanch, 1999). The same account applies to the Federation of American Health Systems, a lobby group for 1400 for-profit hospitals whose leaders were also persuaded that the best way to escape the cost controls of Medicare was to change the nature of the program's entitlement. For these groups and their industry allies, the argument was straightforward. As long as HCFA was willing to use traditional price control tools to rein in hospital and physician expenditure, the industry faced a concentration of payer power they could not hope to overcome.[14] Vouchers, on the other hand, would limit federal outlays, constituting in effect a Medicare global budget. But, unlike Medicare historically, a voucher system would shift the risk of additional spending to beneficiaries and the plans they chose. This is not the place to discuss the substantive policy issues raised by vouchers, topics that at this writing have not been adequately addressed (see Marmor and Oberlander, 1998; Kuttner, 1999). But it is clear that the theoretical appeal of a managed competition plan for Medicare—with vouchers renamed "premium support"—gained backing by 1997 from Republicans who had once railed against virtually the same policy when Bill Clinton and his task force presented their comprehensive reform proposal in 1993. Yet when the commission cochairmen introduced their plan in the Congress, the hearings that ensued reenacted the very disputes that had stalemated their earlier efforts. Medicare had been on something of a roller coaster for the entire decade of the 1990s and ended on the public agenda, but with nothing approaching a consensus on either the seriousness of its problems or the right remedies for them.

NOTES

1. The increase in public concern over health care was quite dramatic in the early 1990s. Although, as noted, only 3 percent of Americans ranked health care and/or Medicare as the most important issue facing the country in 1991, by 1992 it was 12 percent (Gallup Poll, 1992, 160), and by 1993 the figure had grown to 28 percent (Gallup Poll, 1993, 168).

2. For a comprehensive analysis of the political and programmatic implications of the 1997 Medicare reforms, as well as of the "flip-flop" in Medicare politics between 1995 and 1997, see Oberlander (1998).

3. This recalls the lag between public perception and reality Chapter 7 noted about the implementation of DRGs; crisis talk continued at the very time the rate of medical inflation declined.

4. As already noted, the Clinton administration did incorporate cost reductions in Medicare as part of its *fiscal* strategy. Those reductions were less than proposed by the Bush administration and not overtly identified as an objective for the Medicare program.

5. Another analogy is useful here. When the United States declares war, no one shouts that the Department of Defense is going to run out of money. There is, of course, debate over the wisdom of the military engagement and disputes over the willingness of Congress to pay for the additional war-related expenses. However, no one would contend that the increased expenses due to a new military engagement will cause DOD to become bankrupt.

6. The 1995 Trustee Report concluded its gloomy assessment of the Hospital Insurance Trust Fund's short-term and long-term prospects by stating: "We strongly recommend that the crisis presented by the financial condition of the Medicare Trust Funds be urgently addressed on a comprehensive basis, including a review of the programs financing methods, benefits provisions, and delivery mechanisms" (Rushefsky and Patel, 1998, 45).

7. Although the Contract with America did not address health care per se,

the congressional Republicans turned their sights on Medicare to secure the tax and spending cuts promised in the contract (Skocpol, 1997). The House proposed a budget resolution with $288 billion in savings from Medicare for FY 1996–2002 (Rushefsky and Patel, 1998, 116–117).

8.   There was some factual basis for the concern. Certainly the number of retirees is expected to rise significantly, which in turn would put more financial pressure on the Medicare system. However, the affordability of social insurance programs in the future must also take into account the overall ratio of workers to nonworkers (both those under 18 and those retired). That ratio will, according to current estimates, remain relatively constant between the 1990s and 2020, rising to a level through 2040 that is still below the dependency ratio America experienced in 1960 (National Academy on an Aging Society, 1999, 12).

9.   Only 7 million (out of 39 million) recipients had enrolled in HMOs as of the spring of 1999 (*New York Times*, 1998).

10.   Yet HMO enrollment only grew to 6 million out of the 39 million Medicare recipients by the spring of 1999, while Medicare Savings Accounts were little used and none of the other types of private plans were even available (*New York Times,* 1999). In 1997, the CBO projected 1999 enrollment levels in HMOs to have grown much faster, to 7.3 million, and enrollment levels in other types of private plans at close to one million (Congressional Budget Office, 1997, 1, 2).

11.   Although the advocates of Medicare + Choice were vocal supporters of free markets as a means to control costs, in fact Medicare + Choice operated by setting fixed payment per Medicare enrollee at 90 percent of the average cost. Thus, in fact, the savings were by capitation, not by competition per se.

12.   See Notes 9 and 10.

13.   This appearance of mutual gain understates the Republican victories on other features of the Medicare struggles. As Mark Peterson writes, the GOP may have lost its bid to recapture the presidency and suffered some losses in the House in 1996, but it transformed the agenda, altered the terms of debate, and helped unleash a private sector transformation of the health domain that is entirely consistent with its long-term political project of balancing the federal budget, reducing federal spending, and promoting the activist market in place of the activist state. Market-oriented approaches to health care—now even embedded in Medicare, the Democratic bastion of social policy—have distinct winners who reap the rewards of the redistribution of resources they generate. It is the Republican base—business, insurers, some health care providers, pharmaceuticals, movement conservatives, all of the members of the erstwhile No Name Coalition—that has profited from this transformation (Peterson, 1998).

14.   There was growing evidence by the fall of 1998 that in fact HCFA had so effectively controlled payments to HMOs for care of Medicare beneficiaries that HMOs began dropping Medicare patients entirely, claiming that the government premium payments were too low. See, e.g., the *Baltimore Sun* (September 23, 1998), noting Prudential's decision to withdraw from the Medicare markets of Maryland, California, Washington, D.C., New York, New Jersey, and parts of Florida.

9

The Ideological Context of Medicare's Politics

The Presumptions of Medicare's Founders versus the Rise of Procompetitive Ideas in Medical Care

INTRODUCTION

A t the close of the twentieth century, Medicare was at the top of the national political agenda, but without any clear resolution as to whether it would be changed dramatically, adjusted incrementally, or stalemated politically (Kaiser Family Foundation, 1999). The combination of the demands of the presidential race of 2000, the partisan split between the Congress and the Clinton administration, and the ordinary structural constraints of American politics—all made the immediate future unclear and longer-term predictions uncertain. What the conflict was about, however, was somewhat clearer. It was a dispute between those who wanted Medicare to remain largely within the confines of the social insurance model of its birth and those who advocated turning the program into a voucher scheme. The traditional defenders of Medicare sought to shore up its financial future by committing projected federal surpluses to the program. By contrast, the voucher proponents (using the vocabulary of "premium support") presumed that having Medicare beneficiaries choose among competing health insurance plans was the right course of remedial action.

These two visions of Medicare's future rest on profoundly different conceptions of the responsibilities and capacities of government, especially the federal government. They reflect currents of thought that, while relevant to Medicare, are about topics much broader than health insurance for the elderly and the disabled. Consequently, I want here to explore first what happened to the idea of Medicare as the first step to universal health insurance and therefore what conceptions of social insurance are available to bolster the program as it is and as it might be expanded. Second, I will turn to trying to understand how and why the development of procompetitive ideas for public policy came to play such an important role in Medicare debates during the last half of the 1990s and will in all likelihood be set against the "traditional" Medicare assumptions in the years to come.

I.   MEDICARE'S PHILOSOPHICAL ROOTS: SOCIAL INSURANCE AND THE PRESUMPTION OF EXPANSION[1]

The striking fact about the origins of Medicare is not the surprising character of the 1965 program, but the uncertain commitment in the first place to a program for the aged. Health insurance for the aged under Social Security was what reformers thought they could extract from the American politics of the period, not what they ultimately wanted. Medicare proposals thus began with hospital insurance for the elderly, not with the benefits they ought to (or in the end did) include. Protection from the unbudgetable expenses of illness was the announced aim of the Medicare program, but few of its backers imagined that the program features of 1965 constituted reasonable provision of that protection (Bowler, 1987). Rather, in the context of the Great Society's aspirations, the legislation of 1965 was but a first step in a series of pragmatic efforts to make medical care universally accessible and its costs more fairly and sensibly distributed across groups, redistributing the financial burdens from the sick to the well and the poorer to wealthier through social insurance taxes.

Appropriate standards of access and distribution of costs are not, however, directly confronted in incremental, pragmatic adjustments to the political possibilities of the moment. Medicare's philosophical underpinnings—to the extent they were clear in 1965—were largely negative, specification of what Medicare was not rather than what its aims and methods fully entailed. So, for instance, Medicare was not to be like the National Health Service of Great Britain, in which medical care is removed from the market and directly provided by public authorities and their contractual agents. That would have been "socialized medicine" for the old, a negative stereotype self-consciously rejected by Medicare's reformers. Nor was Medicare to be "charity" or welfare medicine. Its immediate predecessor—the Kerr-Mills program enacted in 1960—was precisely that and accordingly judged a great failure (see pages 27–30). Thus, if medical care was to be understood as a merit good and if means-tested programs to assure its availability were unacceptable, it stood to reason that some other form of government intervention into the medical economy was required.

The structure of Medicare as enacted—Social Security financing and eligibility for hospital care (Part A), and premiums plus general revenues for physician expenses (Part B)—had a clear political explanation, not a clearly understood social insurance rationale. The rhetoric was there, but the public's understanding of the distinctions between social and private health insurance was never deep. Moreover, the structure of the benefits themselves, providing acute hospital care and intermittent physician treatment, was not tightly linked to the special circumstances of the elderly as a group. Left out were provisions that addressed the particular problems of the chronically sick elderly: medical conditions that would not dramatically improve and the need to maintain independent function rather than triumph over discrete illness and injury. Viewed as a first step toward universal health insurance, the Medicare strategy made what seemed like obvious sense. But after more than three decades, with essentially no serious restructuring of the benefits, Medicare appeared by the mid-1990s philosophically somewhat ungrounded and practically in need of serious adjustment. (Notably, the program as enacted did *not* cover the cost of prescription drugs. This omission would become a major factor in the calls for Medicare reform at the end of the 1990s.)

Beyond the continuing mismatch between Medicare's benefits and the health circumstances of many of the elderly, there was the unresolved question of what kind of entitlement to medical care Medicare did express. Medicare's social-insurance premises did provide a general basis for a statutory "right" to health insurance coverage. But neither the program's reformers nor subsequent defenders have defined precisely the character of that right or the extent of protection it promised. It is here that the absence of a guiding Medicare philosophy is most apparent. One interpretation of the right to medical care emphasizes, for example, equality of opportunity. For the elderly, circumstances of income, housing, illness, and family all differ, sometimes profoundly. Protection from medical-care expenses, from this point of view, would simply mean that equally ill elderly would receive the same treatment, that their ability to pay for care would be irrelevant to the treatment deemed appropriate. Note that this conception does not require heroic treatment of any particular class of ailments; it requires instead that whatever treatment is otherwise appropriate be provided free of the impediments of class, regions, race, and the like. Equal opportunity in this context means equal treatment, not luxurious treatment, heroic treatment, or unlimited treatment. Ascetic equality is as justifiable as luxurious equality of treatment might be. Considerations other than equality of opportunity would bear on the extent of treatment equally available.

Medicare's development has not reflected a clear commitment to this egalitarian conception of the right to medical care. Were it the dominant conception, the United States might well have followed Canada's example and discouraged the independent insuring of medical expenses that Medicare does not bear (Evans, 1986, 19–24; Marmor and Klein, 1986, 25–34). Consider, for instance, the way supplementary insurance for the elderly developed. Medicare began with a variety of cost-sharing devices to restrain use, a policy that, in the absence of supplementary insurance, redistributes some of the costs of care to the ill among the elderly. Medicare, as noted earlier, has a hospital deductible approximating the average cost of one day of American hospital care, and a deductible for physician services as well as a coinsurance rate of 20 percent on charges Medicare deems "reasonable." Yet, since the incomes of the elderly are unequal, the imposition of equal dollar deductibles or coinsurance in and of itself entails unequal burdens on differently situated older Americans. But this situation was compounded by the 1965 decision to permit supplementary insurance to cover these and other medical expenses. These tax-subsidized insurance policies pay for care Medicare does not finance—like prescription drugs outside the hospital. They also typically pay for Medicare's deductibles and coinsurance, but do so in ways that further complicate the lives of the sick elderly. Over half Medicare's beneficiaries had purchased such coverage by the mid-1980s, with the uncovered disproportionately located among lower-income older Americans (Davis, 1985, 50). As a consequence of this, older Americans face quite different net prices for the care of similar medical conditions. An equal right to health care, properly understood, would proscribe such differences in financing (Marmor and Morone, 1983). A policy that expressed such an understanding would either bar the purchase of insurance protection for expenses Medicare does not cover or pay completely for the care deemed medically necessary and fiscally sensible. The degree to which such reflections have been absent from the deliberations about Medicare helps to explain why, when transformative changes were suggested in the 1990s, the conversations were so confusing, so unsettled. For some, breaking up the risk pool of Medicare violated social insurance principles; for others it is simply a technique for managing public subsidy of health insurance for a particular population group (White, 1998).

Another profound question left unsettled in Medicare debates has been whether the program should finance all the medical care passing the test of efficacy. In the 1980s and 1990s, a number of commentators complained that Medicare's rising outlays unfairly taxed the current working population to produce unwarranted benefits to the contemporary (and often financially comfortable) old. In common language this was the Medicare version of the alleged "generational inequity" of America's social policy toward the elderly. This set of claims raises a number of different issues, only one of which is the topic of reflection here. The most controversial question is whether there are grounds for restricting the care available, even if efficacious and sensible on cost-benefit grounds for the elderly, because of alternative uses of those same funds for other Americans.

This issue highlights claims of generational unfairness that became more prominent as fears about the affordability of an aging population became more widely disseminated in the early 1980s and then again in the late 1990s. Because Medicare (and Social Security) have always enjoyed broad (if not deeply informed) public approval, many critics shifted to complaints that these popular programs can be neither afforded nor managed. That led some thoughtful defenders of Medicare to consider what acceptable constraints on benefits for the elderly might be. Could one, for example, justify the deprivation of effective care for the elderly in a way the elderly themselves might view as just?

Norman Daniels provided an approach to this question in the late 1980s that illuminated the issues at stake (Daniels, 1988). If one pits the care of an older person against that of a younger one, the calculation compares the "utility" of one person to another. This formulation—the interpersonal comparison of utility—is fraught with difficulties no social philosopher has solved. But were the question posed differently—comparing benefits over one individual's lifetime—a reasonable case can be made for concentrating more resources earlier rather than later in life. If the right to health care is understood as the right to return to functioning after illness so as to complete one's plan of life, then a more completed life calls for less expenditure—holding illness constant—than a less completed one. The claims of the 50-year-old, on this account, dominate the claims of the same person at 80 and do so for reasons intelligible to that person. It is as if one were allocating resources over one's lifetime and embodying in that decision a social contract: the older the citizen, the greater the restraint.

This formulation made a genuine contribution to our debate over the allocation of resources for different age groups. It differs from the formulation of generational conflicts in an important respect. The policy of restraint applies not to others, but to oneself at a point in the life cycle. The basis is not the gains to us as opposed to the losses of others, but the distribution of care to us over time. It is hard to imagine a more important philosophical contribution to debates over Medicare than this distinction between the fair treatment of age and the fair treatment of generations. The treatment of generations takes the accidents of the timing of one's birth to decide who gains and who loses, the very essence of arbitrariness in social policy. The fair treatment of aging—a matter in which all are involved similarly—removes this arbitrariness. Nevertheless, there was a crucial limit on the contribution of such thinking to policy debates over Medicare.

The elaboration about what a just distribution of medical care resources requires—important as it is for the justification of universal health insurance—can do little to contribute distinctively to a philosophical rationale for Medicare. There was a strategic reason to start government health insurance with aged beneficiaries of Social Security. There was an incremental rationale for extending coverage in the 1970s to those eligible for the Social Security's disability program and those suffering from renal failure (ESRD). But that provides neither the grounds for universal coverage nor the special reasons why the elderly should enjoy insurance coverage that other equally threatened citizens find impossible to find or afford.

In addition, the special circumstances of Medicare's enactment further undermined the staying power that social insurance principles have displayed, for example, in retirement pensions. From the very beginning, the separate and distinctive financing of Part B benefits—drawn from premiums paid voluntarily (though heavily subsidized) and general revenues—blurred Medicare's link to traditional social insurance sources of revenue. Had Medicare been universalized, the rationalization of its finance would have been more salient. As it happened, the range of financing arrangements gave every theory of public finance a claim on characterizing Medicare. And that in turn meant there was no single compelling characterization with which to resist alterations or to justify expansion.

There was an organizational counterpart to the waning clarity of Medicare's initial rationale. By that I mean the 1977 shift of Medicare's administration from the Social Security Administration to a newly constituted Health Care Financing Agency. As noted earlier, this move seemed to move Medicare away from its social insurance roots and, at the same time, meant that local offices of the Social Security Administration no longer represented Medicare nor monitored its complexities. In addition, the creation of a comprehensive federal agency reflected the prediction that universal health insurance was to happen and the federal role in medical care finance should be consolidated. That was, of course, neither the first nor the last time that the conceptions of Medicare adjustments were dominated by ambitious notions of what the larger role of federal health policy would be.

Conceived as a prelude to national health insurance for all, Medicare became one of America's largest social programs, directing enormous medical resources to the elderly and their providers. But Medicare did not, for a variety of reasons, adjust its benefits to the most distinctive medical circumstances of that group: namely, chronic ailments. With all the attention to the future fiscal problems of Medicare in budget debates since the early 1980s, it is particularly noteworthy that there has been relatively little sustained attention to justifying the care the program does and does not finance.

No such discussion took place when the debate over Medicare returned to the center stage of American politics in the 1995–99 period. Instead, what transpired was a fiscal and ideological dialogue that mixed fact with fiction, fear with claimed prudence, and fantasy with sobriety about the future. The result was a debate in 1998–99 that was as detached from the realities of Medicare and the wants of its beneficiaries as was the debate of 1965 from the understandings of most Americans about what benefits the original legislation covered. In part this gap reflected the absence in America of a guiding philosophy about the proper role of government in medical care, especially an articulation of what health coverage under social insurance required. The lack of clarity became increasingly important as fiscal politics made Medicare's future fearful with forecasts of unaffordability. Viewed this way, understanding Medicare's fundamental presumptions—then and now—is a necessary but not sufficient prerequisite for anticipating its possible futures. Unless its social insurance roots are reinvigorated, Medicare's programmatic operation will continue to come under pressure to resemble the health insurance practices faced by most citizens. That world was, by the end of the twentieth century, one of competition among managed care plans whose private regulation of patients and providers had already alienated a majority of Americans.[2]

II. THE RISE OF PROCOMPETITIVE IDEAS ABOUT MEDICAL CARE

We have already seen how Medicare's enactment represented an initial strategic step toward universal health insurance under social insurance premises. But the premises were not tightly bound to Medicare's administrative features as they developed, and over time the philosophical debates over American medicine largely ignored Medicare. As a result, whatever image of Medicare's incremental expansion there was at the outset increasingly lost its force, as the early reformers aged and the understanding of what social insurance required waned. In the quarter century from the stagflation of the 1970s to the economic boom of the 1990s, another set of ideas reshaped the ideological context in which Medicare's political battles were fought. Commonly described as the rise of a procompetitive ethos, this family of notions depended on a set of dichotomies: markets over governments, competition over regulation, individual choice over collective security. However misleading these simple formulations, they became crucial elements of the external environment setting the terms of the debates over Medicare.

Medicare and the Procompetitive Movement

From our perspective at the end of the twentieth century, it might seem obvious that the debate over Medicare reform should focus on topics like managed care, competitive health plans, and privatization. Such an idea, however, would have been unthinkable at the time of Medicare's enactment in the mid-1960s. For the quarter century after the Second World War, American medicine experienced a golden age of expansion: in scientific research, in the growth of medical institutions, and in the vigorous efforts to distribute these gains more widely in reforms of the 1960s like Medicare, Medicaid, and the community mental health movement.

In the early 1970s the debates about American medicine shifted in a number of important ways. Claims of "crisis" became commonplace as stagflation strained American public budgets, as medical care costs continued to escalate faster than general prices, and as the uninsured again received prominent attention. The language of dismay eclipsed the former, celebratory rhetoric. A sense of urgency marked the atmosphere of medical care debates then, as political elites competed in designing remedies for a medical world that suddenly seemed too costly, too complex, and too callous in an era of rapid inflation and with a growing number of uninsured. It is worth remembering as well that at this time it was assumed the necessary tools of reform would be more extensive governmental planning and more vigorous regulation of the costs of care, the quality of clinical practice, and the location and scale of capital investment.

By the end of 1970s, however, this reformist perspective had been discredited and debunked by many. To promarket critics, the answer to America's medical woes was less regulation, not more, and competitive reforms became a dominant feature of policy debates about American medicine generally (Marmor, 1990). Although Medicare was largely insulated in the 1980s from these newer ideological currents, the genesis of those procompetitive ideas and how they came to be applied to American medicine proved to be crucial to Medicare's fate in the late 1990s and will be important beyond that. With these considerations in mind, we now turn to the rise of procompetitive ideas in American medicine over the last quarter of the twentieth century and its likely bearing on debates in the opening decade of the next century.

At least three factors made the increased attention to competitive ideas an understandable development in the 1970s. First, traditional concerns about access to medical care and the distribution of its costs began to take a back seat to worries about controlling the costs of care—to federal programs, to employers, and so on. Problems of the uninsured and poorly protected could not compete for the public's attention with the genuinely ominous numbers on medical inflation. In 1970, the United States, possessing a strong and growing economy, spent 7.4 percent of its GNP on health care (U.S. Bureau of the Census, 1990, 92). In 1980, with a weak economy still reeling from the twin oil shocks of the previous decade, the proportion was 9.1 percent (ibid.). By 1991, medical care absorbed 11 percent of the GNP and by the end of the decade the United States was spending about 14 percent (*New York Times,* December 30, 1991).

A second factor was the general ascendance in academic writing of a particular microeconomic approach to analyzing public policy, or more accurately, the ascendance of economic analysis that had a deregulatory mission.[3] The antigovernment, free market enthusiasms of economists identified with the University of Chicago conventionally represent this development, but others who would hardly be associated with that movement, like Brookings economist Charles Schultze, were also influential (Melhado, 1988, 145). Indeed, it is fair to say that the neoclassical training of most American economists of this period made the growth of economic analyses of public policy a factor in this assumptive shift. All of this provided the intellectual groundwork for making procompetitive reforms more plausible in medical care.[4]

A third factor bolstering the so-called competitive movement was the spread of the antigovernment, antiregulatory sentiment to the wider political arena. Although for many this movement is synonymous with Ronald Reagan's presidency, it in fact had earlier roots. Richard Nixon's two presidential victories celebrated the limits of government and appeal of market competition even if his administration's domestic policy actions actually expanded federal social policy significantly. American commentators often forget the extent to which Jimmy Carter ran for president on an anti-Washington, antigovernment platform, portraying himself as a down-home farmer who, with pitchfork in hand, was headed to the nation's capital to slay the federal leviathan. The increased legitimacy of this general political ideology—most obviously consequential in traditional areas of governmental regulation like trucking, airlines, and finance—made its application to medical care less problematic than would have been the case at the time of Medicare's birth.

The procompetitive ideology that arose out of the ashes of the 1970s came to have considerable political and rhetorical appeal. The simplest version of the "competitive" answer to social problems was that all public institutions needed to be restructured to accommodate market incentives. The most zealous proponents of competition in medical care confidently claimed that a return to the market would lead to a more sensible control of costs, a more equitable allocation of scarce medical resources, the creation of a more rational delivery system, and the delivery of more appropriate (and perhaps better) medical care. The acceptability of these procompetitive presumptions had become broad enough by 1980 that the *Report of the President's Commission for a National Agenda for the Eighties* could un-self-consciously assert:

> An expansion of the role of competition, consumer choice, and market incentives rather than government control is more likely to create the much needed stimulus toward greater efficiency, cost consciousness, and responsiveness to consumer preferences so visibly lacking in our present arrangements for providing medical care (President's Commission for a National Agenda for the Eighties, 1990, 78–79).

Similar claims received widespread coverage in trade journals, in the popular press, and on Capitol Hill.[5]

The positions advanced under the label of procompetitive were, in fact, diverse and distinguishable. They varied in the degree of change proposed for American medicine, the rationale for such change, and their mechanisms, implementability, and effects. At the same time, while quite separable threads of procompetitive logic ran through these positions, there were some connections among the different proposals. Most importantly, the common ideological appeal to the wonders of markets and competition blurred the substantial differences among three distinct conceptions of how the medical care market should be more competitive.

The view that emerged first in the 1970s emphasized that patients should pay more of their medical bills and face the economic consequences of their consumption decisions. These advocates of "consumer sovereignty" believed that the absence of significant patient cost-sharing in health insurance was the major problem in American medical care. Nearly complete prepayment for care removes the necessity for both the consumer (patient) and the provider (doctor, hospital) to make trade-offs among different medical services and between medical care and other desired economic goods. Even if the consumer were not fully at risk for the cost of medical care, according to this line of argument, the use of deductibles, coinsurance, and copayment would lead consumers to select more economically appropriate forms of care. In short, if the consumer is the best guide to what is desirable and affordable, medical care requires patients to pay. This was an extension—and intensification—of the traditional health insurance rationale for patient cost-sharing. The appeal of this view was expressed in "catastrophic" national health insurance plans of the early 1970s—especially the Long-Ribicoff plan of 1973 and the proposals brought forward under the major risk insurance (MRI) label (Feder, Holahan, and Marmor, 1980). Ironically, this conception of universal catastrophic health insurance—with substantial cost-sharing—had little or no connection to the similarly labeled Medicare legislation of 1987–88.

The second competitive approach was more organizational in emphasis. Advocates of this approach took for granted that American medicine provided too few acceptable alternatives to fee-for-service payment and decentralized medical practices. Of course, medical competition had always existed within what came to be called fee-for-service (FFS) medicine. But that competition was not primarily between conventional practice and the alternative delivery and financing models, such as the prepaid group practices (like Kaiser Permanente), that these reformers would have preferred. By the early 1970s, they had jettisoned the traditional group practice language to distance themselves from its leftwing associations. With the instinct of advertising copywriters, reformers like Dr. Paul Ellwood renamed prepaid group practices as "health maintenance organizations" (HMOs). Promoted by Ellwood energetically, sold to the Nixon administration as an acceptable Republican reform, and popularized in policy circles by Professor Alain Enthoven, the procompetitive HMO movement of the 1970s and 1980s had in mind national health reform, not Medicare's overhaul. Once again, the irony is that the Medicare agenda for the 1990s lagged two decades behind the procompetitive model proposed for American medicine generally.

The proponents of the third view advocated aggressive antitrust rule making, and mobilization to reduce the market power of medical providers. While the other reformers assumed the restructuring of financial systems and altering of reimbursement methods to allow competition on the basis of price, the advocates of antitrust had a somewhat different conception of the primary problem. They contended that collusive behavior on the part of established medical providers prevented the emergence of price competition in the market for medical care. Antitrust law, if enacted, would place a singular emphasis on the benefits of competition. The antitrust preference for competition above any other goal implied that any cost-containing effects of physician or medical system organization would be rejected if the effects were brought about through a lack of competition or by the domination of the market by a particular group.

These were the three broad conceptions of a procompetitive medical care market and, as noted above, they were not necessarily independent of each other. Antitrust action could be used to eliminate barriers to the development of competing groups of medical professionals, a result compatible with the provider reorganization approach. The cost-sharing approach might well permit indemnity insurance with fee-for-service reimbursement to compete with the insurance prices of prepaid group practice. These instrumental connections, however, were less important than the ideological commonalities to which the proponents appealed.

All three procompetitive proposals rejected governmental regulation in the abstract and espoused "correcting" the market they so admired. Procompetitive advocates carefully chose their label, in part to draw an explicit contrast with earlier reform approaches that relied on direct government provision of health insurance. The implication was that other reform proposals were anticompetitive and proregulation. Much of the intuitive appeal of procompetitive proposals was that they represented a form of autoregulation, the suggestion that the "invisible hand" would sort out the allocation of medical care without the heavy hand of public regulation and management.[6] The fact that a system of competing health insurance plans requires extensive regulation to work never received the attention it deserved in this period. And that in turn helps to explain why, over time, the disputes in American medicine pitted idealized models of market transactions against portrayals of actual governmental programs, warts and all. This would be obvious in the late 1990s in the suggestion of the Bipartisan Commission on the Future of Medicare that vouchers and other market devices would right the wrongs of the Medicare program in the twenty-first century.

Market Talk and Medical Care:
The Impact on the Profession and the Public

Not only was there a perceptible increase since the 1970s in the attention paid to proposals to make American medicine more competitive, but a dramatic shift simultaneously took place in the language of medical commentary that will continue to affect the discussion of medical care reform in the future. The traditional doctor-patient relationship becomes, in competitive talk, provider-consumer, or buyer-seller, or supplier-demander. Medicine becomes just another business. The fallout from this refashioned language came to be a threat to the professional ethos of American medicine and by the 1990s had altered the balance of presumption about what to expect from doctors, hospitals, and health insurance.

Traditionally, much of the "income" doctors, nurses and other medical practitioners earned was noneconomic: self-esteem, respect from the community, and idealization as selfless professionals. In casting medical care as no different from other industries, medical professionals were reconceptualized. They no longer deserved (and increasingly no longer received) the noneconomic benefits of public esteem, deferential patients, and the gratitude of families. The stereotype of the medical professional as a self-interested (selfish) agent of business fed on itself. And, over the period under review here (1966–90), the public's esteem for medical practitioners indeed fell sharply (Stevens, 1989, 341–42).

Part of the decreased satisfaction with American medicine undoubtedly arose from worries over costs. Although it is impossible to establish a clear causal connection between the demystification of the medical profession and the increased costs of doctors, the phenomena went hand in hand. For example, despite sharp increases in the number of new physicians, doctors' incomes grew by 30 percent from 1984 to 1989. [This contrasted with an average 16.3 percent increase for other full-time workers over the same period (Fuchs, 1990).] Physicians' fees for procedures were approximately 234 percent higher in the United States than in Canada (Fuchs and Hahn, 1990), and their take-home pay was more than 50 percent higher than that received by Canadian doctors (Evans et al., 1989). It should not be surprising that to the extent professional medical work was increasingly regarded as ordinary commercial activity, higher physician fees (and incomes) were increasingly understood as the result of market power or greed rather than a professional's just desserts.

Patient dissatisfaction begat doctor dissatisfaction. Despite the increase in incomes, the prestige of the medical profession decreased over the 1970s and 1980s. Doctors complained that they no longer enjoyed the autonomy they once had. Rather, elaborate and expensive procedures including utilization reviews, requirements for preadmission certification, and other forms of second-guessing proliferated. One AMA survey in 1986, for example, found that 60 percent of physicians strongly opposed third-party reviews of their hospitalization decisions (Harvey, 1986). In an often-quoted 1991 article in the *Atlantic*, Regina Herzlinger reported that more than 30 percent of current physicians said they would not have attended medical school had they known what their futures had in store (1991, 71).

The language of industrial economics and competitive markets did not just affect doctors. Hospitals and hospital administrators recast themselves in new terms. The hospital administrator increasingly became the chief executive officer. Assistant administrators were refashioned as vice-presidents for their respective functions. These changes were not merely semantic exercises. Rather, they represented a fateful change in the way Americans were encouraged to think of medical care (Marmor, 1998b). The vision of a hospital as primarily a corporate organization—and the concomitant shift in administrative power away from medical staff and toward professional managers— has inevitably affected the way Americans regard medical care. It would be wrong to assume unanimity on this and equally wrong to presume that American physicians and nurses think of themselves simply as business figures. The point here is narrower. Over time, the attack on the professional standing of medicine helped to deflate public confidence and to increase the probability of proposals threatening professional autonomy.

As hospital administrators gave way to chief executive officers (CEOs), so too did their incomes change. By 1990, hospital CEOs earned an average base salary of over $163,000: those receiving incentive pay averaged an additional $125,000. Note that the salaries of these chief administrators increased by 8.5 percent (on average) in 1989, while the Consumer Price Index grew by 4.6 percent (Herzlinger, 1991, 74). And this took place in the midst of a supposed "crisis" in health spending.

There are, of course, advantages to treating medical institutions like hospitals as businesses. Improved capital budgeting and financial and accounting systems are all vital in getting better value for health expenditures. Nor can one pretend medical practitioners are all selfless workers concerned only for the welfare of their patients. Clearly economic motives are important. Indeed, many of the concerns of those who subscribe to procompetitive strategies are identical to those of traditional social insurance advocates. Asymmetries of information and bargaining strength between doctors and patients require attention no matter what the context. Likewise, whatever one's personal philosophy of entitlement to medical care, uncertainty about the efficacy of alternative treatments and the problems of moral hazard and adverse selection all need to be addressed.

But the rhetoric of the competitive reform helped to disguise what sets medicine apart from other industries and it was that broader development in part that made it possible for a Democratic president like Bill Clinton to marry ideas of universal health insurance to "pro-market" ideology, as the preceding chapter noted. That in turn would have consequences for Medicare that were not even dimly imagined in the early 1990s.

In arguing against government-financed or -provided medical care, procompetitive advocates regularly claimed that governments are not sufficiently competent to manage programs like Medicare. The inevitable concessions of the political process made sure, according to this line of argument, that programs in action bear scant resemblance to their initial design. Over time, inefficiency sets in, as governments slowly respond to the results of their actions (which regularly include unintended consequences).

Ironically, procompetitive advocates proposed a variety of detailed government programs, laws, and regulations designed to address and eliminate the "market failures" that occur in any unregulated medical environment. This points to a dilemma that has not been faced in most American discussions of competition in medical care markets. What is one to make of the logic of procompetitive proposals when government incompetence makes impossible the effective reform of medical market failures? How desirable can a plan for "managed competition" be, for example, when only a portion of its provisions get enacted and implemented, when insurance companies are not required to offer specific types of plans, or when the government increases, rather than eliminates, the tax deductibility of medical insurance? What happens if experience rating is allowed (insurers can offer lower premiums to low-risk groups) but the government sets up no provision for high-risk groups who find it difficult to get insurance at all?

The answer is that most procompetitive plans were not robust in precisely this crucial respect—namely, their implementability. They would not perform well unless conditions were just right. By the very detailing of the government actions required to eliminate market failures, advocates of procompetitive reform implicitly acknowledged that without these remedies, competitive systems do not work well. Hence the contradiction in the theory of procompetitive reform. The diagnosis of government failure justifies market reform; the desirability of market competition in health care requires nimble regulation by the very government whose incapacity justifies the appeal to market reform in the first place. Yet, as long as idealized images of market competition were set against operational government programs, the conclusion that market reform was superior proved hard to reject.

The characterization of medical care as just another business also had implications for the way in which the potential for improvement from government intervention came to be judged. The dichotomy drawn between private competition and public regulation invoked free choice and well-functioning markets on the one hand, and the failed socialism of Europe on the other. The dichotomy was (and is) artificial and misleading. The properties of the medical sector are such that regulation of some kind has always been regarded as inevitable by serious writers on the subject. And the most popular "procompetitive" schemes, as noted earlier, all called for a myriad of restrictions on practitioners, payers, and patients alike.

Moreover, what came to be called managed-competition plans in the 1990s presumed the opposite of an unfettered market. On the contrary, these plans required extensive government regulation, indeed a degree of regulation considerably more wide-ranging and complicated than that called for by more traditional national health insurance plans. For example, in the economic struggle among insurance plans encouraged by proponents of managed competition, some firms would have tried to attract young and healthy clients. In rural areas, where it is often difficult to get a single medical provider to cover the population, competition among plans, whatever the encouragement, would have been totally infeasible. To avoid such imbalances, the architects of managed competition designed new organizations to govern the system. Their rules required all citizens to enroll through specified purchasing agents in one or another of a limited number of preapproved plans. For their part, participating insurance companies were required to offer not a single plan, but several predetermined varieties.

But it is not only managed competition that has to be managed. Despite a common procompetitive rhetoric, other reform proposals of the late 1980s and early 1990s presumed an extensive regulatory framework to combat market failures. (Indeed, the language of market failure provided much of the rationale for market reforms.) The plan proposed by the Bush administration, for example, explicitly prohibited health insurance from using experience rating in pricing their policies. A Heritage Foundation proposal, to take another illustration, did not ban experience rating. Instead, it relied on state-regulated and -administered insurance pools to cover high-risk individuals as an alternative instrument to deal with the same problem of unaffordable insurance prices for those with a history of illness (Butler, The Heritage Foundation, 1989).

The legacy of the U.S. debate over medical care reform since the 1970s was twofold. On the one hand, the case for an American version of national health insurance—a Medicare program for all, for example—was weakened. In fact, critics used the problems of American medicine to condemn governmental incapacity. On the other hand, promoters of competition in medicine compared idealized dream worlds with real systems (and, unsurprisingly, ideal systems seemed preferable on paper). To persuade the public of the credibility of the imagined market world, the language of health debates was shrewdly altered. The vocabulary and terminology of economists became the vernacular, and the unquestioning use of this jargon became much more pervasive in debates (Marmor, 1998b).

It was in that context that Bill Clinton came to select managed competition within a global budget as his reform dream. That choice was, as Chapter 8 suggested, fateful and doomed to political controversy. One has to regulate competition in medical care to make it acceptable, but if one does that and increases insurance coverage, the role of government is plain and the attackers have a field day.

In place of national health insurance, the Clinton reform effort left a stalemated political outcome—symbolized by the literal disappearance of the Clinton plan in September 1994—followed by an unprecedented pace of change in American medical care arrangements. Though this is not the place for any extended discussion, it is important for this assessment of the role of competition to note whatever connections there were between the long buildup of competitive ideas and the Clinton debacle.

The resulting story was one of great hopes, great changes, and great disappointment. The hopes of some of the procompetitive advocates—of either consumer sovereignty or organizational reform—were a combination of universal coverage and competitive conditions in the pricing and delivery of medical care. The Clinton reformers also hoped to combine competition in the delivery of care with egalitarian financing of the basic insurance. Their hopes, as we know, were dashed completely. Yet the story was more significant than that. By capturing the interests and energies of so many reform actors, the procompetitive movement siphoned energy away from other strategies of reform in American public life.

The legacy of this rise and transformation of competitive ideas in medical care will be with America for decades. Without the regulation proposed by the Clinton plan, the advocates of what is termed managed competition were set loose. By 1996, 70 percent of Americans were in such plans. Most of those plans managed little else but costs and, in doing so, restricted the choices of both medical professionals and their patients. In the name of expanding choice, American medicine went through a period of extraordinary reduction of choice. Aggregate health costs rose at lower rates in the mid-1990s, but that can be misleading. The ratio of medical care inflation to general inflation, for example, was not markedly reduced. But the rise in costs to American firms did slow for a time, with the externalizing of more costs—both fiscal and psychic—to patients and providers.

Finally, there has been enormous change in the ownership and behavior of insurers, hospitals, medical plans, and drug firms. Organizational consolidation describes much of what has transpired: the growth of multihospital chains like Columbia HCA and the spread to nationwide activities of prepaid group practice organizations like

Kaiser-Permanente. In addition, there was shifting of financial risk—as with carving up capitation payments—and the creation of new firms less to manage medical services than to constrain what care can be given, and reduce or slow the rate of growth in the prices paid.

All of this constitutes an extraordinary set of ironies. In the name of competition, choice narrowed. In the name of consumer responsiveness, consumer complaints shifted in character and increased in anger. In the name of American entrepeneurialism, American physicians turned into employees of firms owned by others. Choice without change, change without choice, this captures the set of ironies. The politics of medicine, as a result, will be increasingly fought out in state legislatures (see Rich and White, 1996). There the disputes are over what degree of public regulation there should be over the enormous amount of private regulation that has already transpired. Very few observers would have predicted the subject of controversy in the state legislatures of the mid-1990s: issues like drive-by mastectomies, limits of one day's hospitalization for the delivery of a child, or gag rules on what doctors could tell their patients about the limits of their managed care plans. Procompetitive enthusiasts did not predict such disputes either, but they have arisen in part because of the role of their ideas in the complicated politics of American medicine.

Since the 1970s there has been a constant and broad dispute over the proper role of government in capitalist democracies. The arguments in favor of increased competition—in medical care generally and particularly within health insurance—received far more favorable responses than at any other time in the period since the Second World War. The United States responded differently to this than other industrial democracies. In Europe the argument for increased competition overwhelmingly took for granted that universal entitlement to health insurance was a given. But American arguments over the role of competition were part of the broader disputes over whether universal health insurance coverage was desirable and implementable. As a result, the story is the rise of procompetitive ideas without a counterpart to the guarantee of insurance coverage.

NOTES

1.   This section follows the analysis in Marmor (1998).

2.   Indeed, by 1999 managed care and health insurers were two of the four industries that less than a majority of Americans said they would trust: tobacco and oil were the others (Harris Poll, 1999).

3.   It may be hard to remember, but at one time economics helped to provide justification for government intervention and regulation. The principal

motive for the increased application of economics to public policy after World War II was the expanding of government as a purveyor of large public programs entailing major expenditures (Melhado, 1988, 35).

4.   Indeed, Melhado cites a personal telephone conversation in which Stanford economist Alain Enthoven reports that he had read Schultze's book, *The Public Use of Private Interest*, shortly before devising his Consumer Choice Health Plan and that he regards his (own) book as the "working out" in the health care economy of an example of Schultze's general propositions (Melhado, 1988, 37).

5.   See, for example, Christianson and McClure (1979) for trade journals and Demkovich (1980) coverage in the popular press and on Capitol Hill.

6.   By "allocate medical care," I mean determine who will get what medical care. The mechanism employed by the market is usually, but not exclusively, price. It is important to note that an often-unstated assumption of procompetitive advocates for health care is that the market itself can not only efficiently, but also *appropriately* allocate care. The support for this normative claim is rarely given.

10

Reflections on Medicare's Politics: Puzzles and Patterns

INTRODUCTION

This chapter sets out analytically what has been suggested—sometimes explicitly, sometimes implicitly—in the preceding chapters. This effort, parallel to what was done in Chapter 5 of Part I, addresses the patterns of Medicare, the puzzles its politics pose, and the types of approaches one needs to make sense of those puzzles. The story of Medicare's operational development since 1966 is marked by both irony and turbulence. The social insurance philosophy that ensured its original appeal as a proposal used the trust fund terminology for Part A to suggest a sense of financial pre-commitment and thus political stability to Medicare. But, over time, forecasts of the trust fund accounting—and projections of 'insolvency'—have partly undermined the very sense of security the trust fund was supposed to engender. The administrative compromises deemed necessary for Medicare's passage in 1965 nonetheless contributed to the subsequent and worrisome inflation in medical care. That development in turn produced effects quite inimical to the expansionist intentions of Medicare's original sponsors. The understanding of these discrepancies, surprises, and disappointments lies not so much in the Byzantine subtleties of legislative bargaining and the idiosyncrasies of political personalities as in the political forces that framed this bargaining and shaped program operations after 1965.

UNDERSTANDING MEDICARE'S POLITICS: PATTERNS, PUZZLES, AND EXPLANATORY APPROACHES

The preceding chapters on Medicare postenactment describe a politics dominated by administrative and fiscal issues. Those politics paid relatively little attention to disputes over the medical needs of the elderly and whether the program was adequately addressing them. Medicare's first five years, from 1966 to 1971, were years of "accommodation" to American medicine in Larry Brown's appropriate phrase. But the smooth and efficient implementation of the program was purchased at the cost of built-in inflationary pressures. In the 1970s, in contrast, there were substantive changes in benefits (for example, to cover dialysis and the disabled). But much more political attention was given to nationwide medical reform. The first puzzle this chapter discusses is not what happened in the 1970s, but whether it might have been different. So, for example, is the explanation for Medicare's limited expansion one of the situational politics of the period? Or are the limits of expansion the result of more powerful, structural factors in the American polity that not only determined the constraints on Medicare but shaped the fate of universal health insurance proposals more generally?

Medicare has always been the subject of intense interest group politics. But concerns about spiraling medical costs and the growing federal deficit increasingly came to the public's attention and shaped political debate over Medicare in the 1980s and 1990s. Indeed, the politics of the federal deficit, it is not too much to claim, dominated Medicare policy debates from 1980 to the enactment of the Medicare reforms of 1997. The second puzzle analyzed in this chapter, then, is what explains this evident pattern of fiscal politics and the recurrent "crises" we have already described. And how can the regulatory programs that emerged—from administered prices in the hospital industry to tightened fee schedules for physicians—be reconciled with the procompetitive ideology of the Reagan-Bush administrations?

The struggles over Medicare in the 1990s, as Chapter 8 noted, were shaped by a variety of factors. The Clinton administration's effort to implement national health insurance, the shift in partisan control of the Congress in 1994, the Presidential election of 1996, and growing fears that the impending retirement of baby boomers would leave Medicare "bankrupt"—all were components of the narrative account. Within that history, however, is a puzzle that calls for explicit analytical attention. Why did the reform ideas associated with the failed Clinton health insurance proposal of 1992–94 reappear as a plausible policy answer for Medicare in the period 1995–99? Why was there a flip-flop—particularly by Republican congressional leaders—over "managed competition" when the topic changed from universal health insurance to the "re-form" of Medicare?

These, then are the puzzles on which I want to reflect, each of which calls forth in my view a quite different type of explanation. A summary of Medicare's politics in the three decades after enactment, however understandable, cannot substitute for a causal account. Put another way, the narrative of what happened cannot answer why those patterns emerged. To do so requires integrating three factors largely implicit in Chapters 7 and 8. One has to do with contemporary interpretations about the state of the economy and political order at any one time and the impact of those beliefs on the definition of Medicare's "problems" and the range of plausible "remedies." Medicare's standard operating procedures—and the accepted organizational ideas they reflected—constitute the second category of causally important factors. And, third, there are the changing distributions of political power within the formal institutions of government, especially shifts in the party affiliation within the Congress and between the Congress and the administration. All three of these causal factors are important: the first to define the problems that were on the political agenda, the second to specify the range of options that were operationally available, and the third to account for what choices were made among the options available to deal with the problems identified. Just as with the explanation for Medicare's enactment, the scholarly explanation for Medicare's political history requires attention to these quite distinguishable levels of analysis.[1]

PUZZLE ONE: STRUCTURAL EXPLANATIONS AND MEDICARE'S LIMITED EVOLUTION

A striking feature of Medicare's evolution since 1965 has been continuity—in basic financing sources, range of benefits, types of regulation, and, less obviously, beneficiaries. Put another way, for a program understood by reform advocates as the first step to universal health insurance, the puzzle is why there has been no dramatic expansion of who is covered or for what medical costs. (By contrast, for example, the politics of expansion in Canada proceeded in two large national steps: universal hospital insurance legislation and implementation, 1957–61, and then physician coverage, 1968–71.) The absence of fundamental expansion does not, of course, mean no change in policy, program operation, or coverage, as Medicare's inclusion in the early 1970s of the disabled and victims of renal failure illustrates. Nonetheless, the limits on expansion require explanation just as does the expansion beyond previous limits.

One approach to why Medicare has been constrained in expansion—and universal health insurance stalemated for most of the twentieth century—is what we have termed a "structural" account of political change (Marmor and Mashaw, 1996, 68 ff.). Structural explanations begin with the constitutional allocation of political authority, which means in the United States the fragmentation of institutional power expressed formally as separation of powers and federalism. This constitutional fragmentation means that large-scale policy change is less likely in the United States, other things equal, than in regimes with more unified political authority. Indeed, something close to super-majorities are required to overcome the legislative gauntlet civics books describe as "how a bill becomes a law." A second structural constraint on political action is the distribution of fundamental beliefs about what government should and should not do. By that I mean not the slogans of particular parties or political contestants, but the underlying, deeper ideological commitments those slogans are meant to engage.

Viewed through this analytical lens, the structure of American politics is one of hobbled majoritarianism. Even where mass preferences appear clear—as with majority support for universal health insurance over most of the decades since the 1930s—the dispersion of authority provides ample opportunity for derailing reform plans. In addition, the underlying ideology of the American public is at best ambivalent about the positive role of government in domestic life. An "enduring unease regarding state interference awkwardly coexists with an acceptance of state involvement in specific social welfare programs" (Jacobs, 1993; Marmor and Mashaw, 1996, 650).

The implication of this structural account should by now be reasonably clear. Medicare's enactment emerged under extraordinary circumstances: a super-majority in the aftermath of the Kennedy assassination and the overwhelming Democratic victories in the presidential and congressional races of 1964. Absent such majorities, one should not be surprised at limits on major change in Medicare—or continued stalemate over universal health insurance coverage either.

There is one counterfactual that might well arise in connection with this structural approach. If super-majorities are both rare in American politics and crucial to explaining major change, did Medicare reformers make a huge mistake in 1965 in limiting their aspirations to what had been on the agenda in less propitious times? Were they, to use the vernacular, "stupid" not to demand more? Should they have tried to make Medicare an instrument to reform American medicine then rather than an adaptation to it? To answer such questions requires attention to the understandings of the participants in the negotiations over Medicare's enactment, details presented in the narrative, but analytically highlighted by what the first edition identified as Allison's model of "bureaucratic politics" (Allison, 1968). The more one understands those reformers, the less "stupid" their choices seem. But, equally, the risk-averse decisions of the 1960s, however comprehensible, were consequential. They rested on presumptions about Medicare's incremental expansion that simply did not turn out to be the case, as Chapter 9 emphasizes.

PUZZLE TWO: INSIDER POLITICS, MEDICARE'S PRICE CONTROLS, AND THE PUZZLES OF THE REAGAN/BUSH ERA

How can one explain the seemingly puzzling fact that in the 1980s presidential administrations committed to a free-market ideology agreed to impose administered prices on American hospitals and physicians? It is certainly not the case that the structural constraints of American constitutional design entailed anything like diagnosis-related group payment for Medicare's hospital bills. Nor are there grounds for believing this was largely circumstantial, a seeming accident of a special, momentary configuration of setting, participants, and interests. Rather, the regulatory pattern of the 1980s emerged over years and has been sustained. Here, the most promising explanatory approach is a hybrid, something in between the constraints of fundamental structures and the momentary alignment of political forces. This is the explanatory approach Chapter 5 characterizes as "organizational"—paying attention to "stable, institutional rules and relationships, the inertial weight of existing arrangements, and ideological commitments that are malleable, but not in the short run" (Graetz and Mashaw, 375).

The existing rules and relationships for Medicare policymaking in the 1980s were those we can call "insider politics." The relevant participants were the congressional committees with jurisdiction, the interest groups most affected by Medicare's payment policies, and the administrative officials in HCFA—all of whom dealt with each other regularly. To the extent the Reagan administration wanted constraints on Medicare's hospital outlays, the range of relevant options—absent a super-majority of Republican legislators—were those acceptable to congressional Democrats in leadership positions, to managers in HCFA, and to significant sectors of the hospital community. The congressional Democrats presumed reliance on Medicare's history of regulating hospital prices. The interest groups had some familiarity with DRGs from experiments in New Jersey. HCFA officials had fostered and indeed financed the experiments that made DRGs an operational option. Without such understanding, Medicare's expansion of prospective reimbursement and tighter fee schedules during the Reagan-Bush era of the 1980s would be truly anomalous. Whether we call this micropolitics or insider politics, the puzzles it resolves are very different from those changes whose explanation demands attention to large-scale changes in the external political environment.

PUZZLE THREE: MEDICARE 1995–99—MACRO POLITICS AND THE EMERGENCE OF UNEXPECTED REMEDIES

A visitor from Canada who observed the fight over the Clinton health reform proposal in the early 1990s would, had she returned in 1995, been surprised by the advocacy of Republican legislative leaders for a system of vouchers in Medicare. Had the visitor stayed on to observe the struggle over the terms of the Balanced Budget Amendments of 1997 and the subsequent deliberations of the National Bipartisan Commission on the Future of Medicare, the puzzle would have deepened. Indeed, the key question might well have been the one raised at the close of Chapter 8: how to explain the flip-flop of previous critics of "managed competition" when the object of reform changed from universal health insurance to Medicare.

My approach to that puzzle is to emphasize the impact of large-scale shifts in the balance of political power within the government. These electoral shifts, in turn, determine what problems are highlighted or subordinated, and what range of remedies is considered feasible or infeasible. Most simply put, the unexpected shift to Republican control of the Congress in 1994, combined with the constraints imposed by the balanced budget politics of 1997, made this flip-flop plausible where it once would have been extraordinary.

There are a number of explanations for the flip-flop that are simply wrong. It was not the case, for example, that public opinion shifted sharply and politicians were feeling pressure to make managed care dominant within Medicare (Aaron and Reischauer, 1995, 1998). If anything, the appeal of managed care within the broader American public had dropped precipitously in the 1995–98 period (Harris Poll, 1999).[2] Note, in addition, that since enactment public opinion has never been a major innovative force in Medicare policymaking. To the extent public opinion has been influential, it has set limits on efforts to transform Medicare, particularly serving to constrain program cutbacks (Oberlander, 1995). Insofar as voucher proposals were an attempt to cut back public benefits indirectly, there was no demand for them from the public. (Public opinion may doom voucher reforms; it did not produce them.)

Nor did electoral shifts in 1998—or changes in the announced positions of the Democratic or Republican parties—play a major role in the demands for a major transformation of Medicare in 1998–99. The other sources of traditional political science explanations offer some limited help here. Interest groups within the medical care industry surely had a role in popularizing both managed care and competitive models of cost control throughout the decade. But that was close to a constant throughout the 1990s; a constant cannot itself explain the unexpected prominence of vouchers in 1998–99.

What can is a complicated (and unplanned) combination of elements, none of which alone would have produced the resultant outcome. Chapter 8 noted the conversion of Republican leaders to a managed competition plan for Medicare, with vouchers renamed "premium support," and the influence exerted by the AMA and the Federation of American Health Systems. To understand this conversion experience requires distinguishing Republican distaste for "big government" initiative (like the Clinton health reform plan) from Republican pragmatism about how to control existing government programs (like Medicare). Vouchers appeal generally to Republicans and, in the case of Medicare, they seemed an acceptable way to reduce federal expenditures in the future and thus to secure the balanced budget that fiscal policy conservatives had long sought (White, 1998). The use of "premium support" as a synonym for vouchers illustrated the search for euphemisms that excited less controversy. Voucher proposals had been notoriously conflictual in the world of public education and the notion of supporting premiums seemed a more neutral expression. The policy idea, nonetheless, was obvious, even if linguistically masked. The theory held that with a fixed sum Medicare beneficiaries would shop for the insurance plan they wanted, with competition among the plans holding down inflation. Relying on that reasoning, advocates projected considerable savings from what Medicare otherwise was projected to spend in the decades after 1998. Then the game shifted to expanding benefits, including most prominently prescription drugs. With cost control predicted, benefits expanded, competition at work, and choice to be enhanced, the conventional claim by the late 1990s was that Medicare would finally be ready for the twenty-first century.

The work during 1998–99 of the 17-member Bipartisan Commission illustrated the rise to prominence of the view that Medicare required transformation. The commission, as noted, disbanded without a formal recommendation. But, within little more than a month, two developments took place. First, the Medicare trustees reported that the hospital account was in much better condition than anyone had predicted just a year before. Medicare's expenses generally rose by only 1.5 percent in 1997–98 and the Part A trust fund would have enough funds to pay its bills until 2015. This was hardly the crisis requiring immediate reform of Medicare and called into question the presumption of unaffordability that had dominated Medicare debates from 1997 to early 1999.

The headlines prior to the commission report's release captured the direction of proposed reform; the *Boston Globe* claimed that "sweeping Medicare overhaul is planned," and that a "free market solution [was] touted to cut costs" (February 28, 1999). The Breaux-Thomas proposal in 1999 that Medicare be transformed into a quite different program conflicted simply with both what public opinion experts would have predicted and commentators within Washington would have thought imaginable in 1993–94. But the suggestion that Medicare requires fundamental alteration is precisely what a substantial proportion of the elite political community contemplated in 1998–99.

What is striking upon reflection is how unsubstantiated were the premises from which the reform proposal proceeded. Medicare was, according to this view, not sustainable in its traditional form. So expensive that it was sure to "run out of money" in time, Medicare was labeled as archaic according to (self-identified) "health care specialists." Seen as "out of touch with modern medical realities," Medicare, for the commission's majority, ought to "harness the power of market competition to lower cost and improve quality of care" (ibid.).

And yet each of these premises conflicted with facts known in 1999 by most Medicare scholars. Medicare was hardly unsustainable in its present form: in 1997–98 its outlays had increased by a mere 1.5 percent and for most of its history its costs had increased no more than the private health insurance plans with which it was being compared. Further, the question of "running out of money" represented an intellectual confusion. As discussed in Chapter 8, it involves the substitution of the thermometer of the trust fund for the causes of genuinely unaffordable outlays. (No one would warn that the Defense Department would become insolvent in discussions of military financing; the notion of insolvency was an artifact of accounting procedures, not an unavoidable feature of the real economy.) Finally, the claim that Medicare was "archaic" represented sheer perversity. The developments in American medicine during the 1990s had made so-called managed care a butt of jokes among ordinary Americans, not a model to be followed. In addition, the claim that managed care could save substantial expenditures was intellectually undermined by the very surge in private insurance outlays in 1998–99. The appeal to the supposed virtues of "managed care" in 1999 was more a function of interest group rhetoric and elite presumptions about interest group power than popular consultation or defensible analysis.

Yet, the conventional competitive strategy for Medicare reform did not constitute an inexplicable anomaly. It was an outcome no one would have expected at the beginning of the decade, but whose lineage is clear with hindsight. Once the Clinton administration embraced "competition" as the right answer to America's medical woes in 1993, the president could not easily reject that "solution" for Medicare when Republican and conservative Democratic legislators embraced it again in 1999. To do so would be to discredit his New Democrat conviction that big government was no longer required and market devices were generally the most effective instruments of public policy. Republican control of Congress after 1994 meant, moreover, that their leaders could be counted on to advance such market solutions.

Just as with the birth of Medicare, the changing partisan composition of the Congress made the crucial difference. Had President Clinton returned for a second term with a Democratic Congress, he would not have been impeached and the Medicare Commission's radical reforms might well have been rejected out of hand. The question for Medicare's future in the spring of 1999 was whether liberal Democrats could persuade the president to reject the reform proposal his own rhetoric had helped to generate. By the fall, they succeeded. What can be claimed with certainty is that the framework for debating Medicare's future was substantially altered once again by the partisan composition of American politics (Peterson, 1999). The question for futurologists is not so much to project Medicare's expenditures or the obvious demographic pressures but to anticipate the varying political responses that different coalitions will make in the first decades of the twenty-first century.

CONCLUSION

Part I examined the politics of Medicare's enactment and answered one particular set of questions. How could the American political system yield a policy that simultaneously appeased widely held antigovernment biases and yet used the federal government to provide a major social insurance entitlement? How was one particularly strong interest group—the AMA—overcome legislatively and yet placated enough to participate in Medicare? Most of all, how did the Medicare law emerge so enlarged from the earlier proposals that themselves had occasioned such controversy? The chapters of Part I explain the rather curious progression by which the primary and strategically narrow aim of "initially" providing federal hospital insurance for the elderly (Part A) was at the last minute substantially expanded, with the approval of former opponents. That 1965 legislative expansion included the separate contributory insurance program for physicians' fees (Part B) as well as state-administered Medicaid, thereby producing what was commonly referred to as an unexpected "three-layer cake." These puzzles of Medicare—the movement from idea to legislation, the surprisingly comprehensive result, and the attendant explanations—belonged to a particular time and a distinctive way of viewing Medicare's enactment politics that Chapter 5 discusses in detail.

The story of Part II is, as the preface noted, quite different. Its subject, the changing politics of Medicare since 1966, is primarily the politics of the program's administration. This altered focus raised a new set of questions about Medicare. Over time, the program became a central element in the political and economic world of American medical care. Through most of its programmatic history Medicare, like American medicine, experienced inflationary pressures beyond everyone's worst fears in 1966. Cost control—in the form of a variety of federal, state, and private sector initiatives that first appeared a few years after Medicare's enactment—regularly disappointed budget officials. Moreover, the place of Medicare in national health politics regularly shifted. National health insurance, so important in the 1970s, largely disappeared from the nation's agenda in the 1980s. And, throughout the period 1966–99, Medicare's fate was shaped as much by broader forces in the political and economic environment as by developments within the narrow medical care domain.

The hopes and expectations engendered by Medicare's passage gave way over time to doubts about the effectiveness of American government and ideological confusion about what Medicare's performance really signified. This was clear by the late 1990s, when Medicare returned to public prominence. What emerged was a largely unapologetic, dynamic, market-oriented medical and political environment— an environment that partly reflected Medicare's disappointments. It was (and is) a medical environment in which too many patients came to be turned away from emergency rooms and sent to beleaguered public hospitals; in which pressures on hospitals encouraged too many doctors to discharge their patients prematurely. It is as well a context in which benefit exclusions, deductibles, and coinsurance have eroded the comprehensiveness of the protection to which Medicare originally aspired and one in which broader questions of patient rights have become prominent. The question in the spring of 1999 was not, "When will national health insurance be enacted?" Rather, for traditional supporters of Medicare, it was, "Can the program retain (or improve on) the gains made in access, security, and equity for the old and, especially, can prescription drugs be added to Medicare's benefits?" And, for the critics, the issue was "how to reform an archaic, unsustainable, Medicare program out of touch with the realities of American medicine?" (*Boston Globe*, February 28, 1999).

It should come as no surprise to the reader that at the end of the twentieth century there remain deep ideological divisions over the pur-

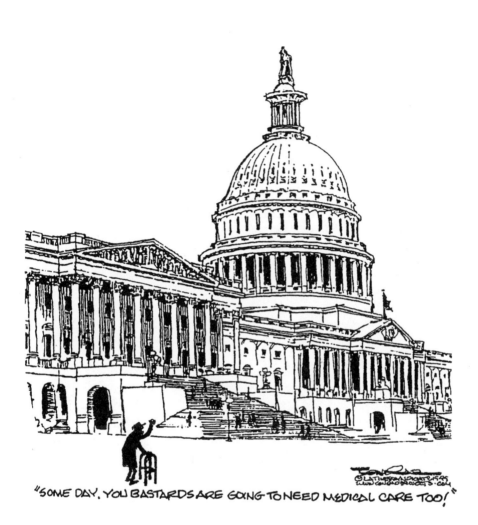

"SOME DAY, YOU BASTARDS ARE GOING TO NEED MEDICAL CARE TOO!"

pose, structure, and future of the Medicare program. As the first edition of this book showed, the critics of Medicare's original formulation were defeated, not converted. The enactment of Medicare came in the wake of a seismic shift in the electorate and a transformation of the congressional balance of partisan power. The puzzles of this final chapter illustrate the interplay of causal influences outside of Medicare and those more closely related to the program's organization and immediate constituencies.

So, for example, there is no understanding the frustrated expansionist ambitions of Medicare's architects without taking into account the impact of the Vietnam war controversies and the stagflation of the 1970s on the evaluation of the Great Society's reforms and the political fate of national health insurance in that period. The Reagan era brought with it not only divided government but also the creation of a fiscal politics that would powerfully (re)shape the overall public policy environment. And, finally, as this chapter has emphasized, understanding Medicare's fate in the 1990s requires attention to the context in which the Clinton administration experienced humiliating defeat over health reform in 1993–94. That context changed substantially through the rest of the decade. With Republican control of the Congress, Democratic control of the White House, and the fiscal orthodoxy of a balanced budget in place by 1997, the options for Medicare's future and their political prospects were bound to alter.

Nonetheless, these options are not simply a matter of reading the bills introduced in recent Congresses. Nor are they simple extrapolations of trends in progress. Rather, as with Medicare's origins, efforts to change the program reflect presumptions about the role of government in American life and the purposes of social insurance in paying for medical care. Medicare's fate will soon be intertwined once again with proposals to expand insurance coverage for the nation. That much the developments in the presidential campaign strategy of Democratic contender Bill Bradley made plain by the fall of 1999. Equally obvious the controversies about "managed care" and whether Medicare should embrace or reject its expansion are on the agenda of American politics. The agenda's range, however, is subject to transformation by both electoral and economic shifts and no one can claim with certainty what the political and economic environment will be like a few years ahead, let alone decades.

What can be concluded, however, is that the politics of Medicare will consist of two types of policy disputes. First, the relatively narrow policy disputes where the ideological cleavages in the larger public are largely irrelevant and second, those relatively rare but important disputes where the deepest divides in the American polity are crucially relevant. That is what the politics of the Medicare program reveals, both in its origins and in its programmatic history.

NOTES

1. It is also useful to analyze Medicare's politics by the program's substantive features. Jon Oberlander has done precisely that, and I have relied in Chapter 8 on his generalizations. Oberlander found three patterns in Medicare policy disputes: struggles over benefits (with a pattern of nondistributive politics), over financing (where the pattern has been one of crisis politics), and over federal payments (where the politics have centered on the budget). Benefits policy means what Medicare does and does not pay for—including long-standing issues of whether prescription drugs and long-term care should be included in the services insured by Parts A and B. Oberlander describes the "pattern" in this area as "non-distributive politics." By that, he means simply that Medicare's development since 1966 has not been one of expansion of benefits, "despite the existence of political incentives that [according to scholars like James Q. Wilson (Wilson, 1973, cited in Oberlander, 1995, 5) might have generated the politics of distribution." To be sure, Medicare came in the 1970s to insure new beneficiaries—victims of renal failure and the disabled under social security. But the generalization still holds. Medicare has not experienced persistent expansion of its health insurance benefits even though those who stand to gain from the program—both insured and providers—have been well- organized to demand expansion.

Second, the "core feature of Medicare financing policy has been crisis politics" (ibid.). What Oberlander means here is that the structure of Medicare's financing arrangements—the sources of funds ranging from payroll taxes to general revenues to beneficiary contributions—has "created recurrent bankruptcy crises," as Chapters 7 and 8 emphasized, prominent, "focusing" events in the program's politics (ibid.).

The third category is Medicare's regulatory politics, the program's policies affecting "payment to medical providers . . . and the medical practices of these providers." The main pattern here, according to Oberlander, "has been budgetary politics" in which the regulation of hospital and physician payments has largely responded to fiscal pressures and become intimately "intertwined with the federal budgetary process." The key generalization is that "crises in Medicare financing explain the timing and political viability of [most] of Medicare's regulatory reforms" (ibid.). This characterization was crucial to Part II's account and highlighted in the reflections of the final chapter.

2. In fact, the public was voicing increasing unhappiness with managed care in the private sector at precisely the same time that Washington began to talk seriously about applying the managed care concept to Medicare (Harris Poll, 1999).

Medicare Scholarship:
A Selective Review Essay

The bibliographical perspective of the first edition of this book was conventional for a young scholar. It lists the books, articles, documents, interviews, and other primary sources on which I depended in writing about the political battle over Medicare's enactment. It is not so much evaluative as revelatory, showing the reader where I looked, what I took to be important, and how I placed the Medicare analysis in the wider scholarship on American politics. In this second edition, I have faithfully reproduced these bibliographical parts (originally entitled "Bibliographical Citations" and "Sources, Acknowledgments, and Further Readings.") This is consistent with my intention to leave the first edition as it was both because future students of Medicare might want to challenge the original interpretation and because that interpretation rested on materials available then, not now.

THE SECOND EDITION: A BIBLIOGRAPHICAL NOTE

The scholarship on Medicare over the period since the first edition was published in 1973 has been voluminous. I will not attempt to characterize its range or quality in detail since that has already been done exhaustively in Jon Oberlander's 1995 thesis, "Medicare and the American State." (Oberlander's bibliography is now available from the University of Michigan's Dissertation Services and will appear in print when his book on Medicare is published.) Instead, I want to cite the major works on which this edition has relied and suggest to the reader what might be helpful on particular topics.

One striking feature of the scholarship on the politics of Medicare's origins and enactment has been the limited attention devoted to reconsidering that episode in the history of the American welfare state. Between 1960 and 1970, a quite substantial number of books was written about the struggle over Medicare. Beyond those cited in the first edition and/or published then—Somers and Somers (1961, 1967), Feingold (1966), Greenfield (1966), Corning (1969), Skidmore (1970), and Harris—only two books have been published since the 1970s that concentrated on the politics of this dramatic innovation in American social policy. One is Sheri David's 1985 account of the history of Medicare and Medicaid's origins (David, 1985). The other is Lawrence Jacobs's 1993 comparative study of the role of public opinion in the enactment of both Medicare and the British National Health Service (Jacobs, 1993).

The scope of the David book is somewhat narrower than that of *The Politics of Medicare*'s first edition. It is a closely detailed, amply footnoted history of congressional treatment of Medicare proposals between 1957 and 1965. Professor David's intent, however, is not reconstruction for its own sake. Rather, as she explains it, it is necessary to "examine the choices, options, and compromises made during the entire Medicare debate . . . before [the nation] can sensibly proceed to solve present and future health care problems" (cited in Marmor, Schlesinger, and Smithey 1986).

David's detailed reconstruction of the congressional fight over Medicare reminds one of the great energies that went into the program's enactment and of the expansionist aspirations of its backers. But it neither challenges the interpretation of *The Politics of Medicare* nor makes a persuasive case that understanding the origins of Medicare is the necessary precondition for righting the wrongs of American medicine. What it does do is provide more facts and information about the congressional handling of Medicare. These are details of who did what, to whom, and when—data that future analysts using Allison's Model III may well want to address in the manner Chapter 5 discusses.

Lawrence Jacobs's book is a different matter. Broadly interested in public opinion's impact on the politics of major healthcare programs, Jacobs addresses the enactment of Medicare as a case example. His major general claim is that "public preferences and understandings have extensive influence on detailed policy making" and he substantiates that argument with extensive primary research on the legislative enactment of both Medicare in 1965 and the British National Health Service in 1946. In short, Jacobs challenges one of the major conclusions of the first edition: the "limited role of mass opinion . . . in this major public policy choice" (Jacobs, 1993, 112). For those interested in the role of mass opinion in the formulation of public policy, Jacobs's book—and his scholarship more generally—should be consulted and the differences in interpretation noted.

Some of Jacobs's findings, however, extend the understandings of the first edition in ways that are important to note. For example, he found conflicts within the executive branch about how Medicare was to be administered. He uncovered a split between the reformers in the Department of Health, Education and Welfare and fiscally cautious leaders in the Bureau of the Budget. The former favored conciliation and accommodation with providers—especially by conceding to private insurance firms the role of fiscal intermediary—so as to make the future road to national health insurance more likely. The latter group— the federal budget officials—regarded the control of expected inflation as the most important concern and thought direct federal administration of Medicare would control costs more reliably. The choice between these two policies marked a victory for HEW's accommodation policy. Chapter 7 notes the importance and implications of that fateful choice, but not the process out of which it emerged. In that way, Jacobs's scholarship reveals a hidden part of Medicare's administrative birth.

Other than these two books, there has been no new, substantial scholarly attention devoted to understanding the origins of Medicare. It is the case that historians of postwar American politics note the program in their accounts, but, other than Sheri David, none has produced a monograph on the topic of which I am aware.

PART II: THE LITERATURE ON MEDICARE'S ADMINISTRATIVE POLITICS, 1966–99

As noted above, there was a good deal of scholarly attention paid in the 1960s and early 1970s to the politics of Medicare's enactment. The same is not true for Medicare's programmatic operation. The overwhelming bulk of scholarly work on Medicare's operations has been in what can be termed the health services research tradition. By that I mean the following. The questions asked by scholars have concentrated on how Medicare has in fact worked (program description), what have been the effects of specific operational policies (program evaluation), and what effects proposed policies might have (policy analysis). In addition to these traditional subjects of policy appraisal, many analysts of Medicare have treated the traditional topics in health economics (the demand for and the supply of services for Medicare) and public health (the epidemiology of aging, the assessment of medical interventions, and so on). There has, in short, been something of a scholarly imbalance, one that has had an important effect on (mis)understandings of Medicare. That, however, is a topic for a separate essay. What follows here is a sketch of those works on Medicare's politics on which I have relied in ways that citations might not fully reveal.

The political analysis of Medicare in operation has been relatively infrequent, almost all article length, and much less connected to the general study of American politics than was the case with the fight over the program's enactment. No comprehensive book-length treatment of Medicare's postenactment politics has been written, though there are two illustrations of near-books. The most extensive is Jon Oberlander's 1995 doctoral dissertation, which will be published in an expanded form within the next few years. As Part II's conclusions and citations illustrate, I have relied considerably on Professor Oberlander's primary scholarship. The second was published in 1999 by Professor Tim Jost of Ohio State's Law School (Jost, 1999). Concentrating on the role of courts in Medicare's history, Jost has produced the most comprehensive published account so far of the forces shaping the politics of Medicare policymaking since 1966. His conclusions are largely compatible with the generalizations of Part II: congressional domination of much of Medicare's policymaking, the salience of fiscal politics in the period since 1983, the relative weakness of public opinion in expanding Medicare's benefits and the relative strength of public opinion in constraining large-scale reductions of benefits. In these respects, the scholarship of Oberlander and Jost complement one another and provided either inspiration or support for the generalizations of Part II's chapters.

There are a number of very helpful accounts of Medicare in the monographic literature on which I have drawn and to which I commend attention. Mark Peterson's writing on the Congress, cited extensively in Chapter 8, is a very good and recent example. While not concentrating on Medicare, Peterson's analysis of what happened to congressional policymaking in the 1990s is especially useful to an understanding of Medicare's political fate in the latter half of the decade. Larry Jacobs's later scholarship on public opinion (Jacobs, 1999) shows how the views of the mass public constrained efforts to restrict Medicare's benefits, but did not otherwise play a major role in affecting Medicare's policymaking in the 1990s. His scholarship is consistent with the contentions of Part II and reinforces the independent, but similar conclusions of Oberlander's work. I should mention as well the article by Larry Brown in the *Health Care Financing Review,* an article that brilliantly distinguishes between the complicated politics of Medicare reform in the 1990s and the relative ease with which analysts describe the "problems" that "need" fixing (Brown, 1996). Brown's earlier article on the "periods" of Medicare's politics provided the initial framework for my discussion of what struggles the program faced over time (Brown, 1985).

It would be wrong to give the impression that no political scientists have written books on Medicare in operation. Rather, the few that have are quite easy to identify. Judy Feder published in 1977 what was then a fresh investigation of how the hospital industry and Medicare had dealt with each other in the Medicare battle, both during the legislative struggle and in Medicare's early years of operation (Feder, 1977). David Smith, writing in the 1980s, took as his central subject the political struggle over paying hospitals that culminated in the widely noticed DRG (Diagnosis-Related Group) reform in 1983 (Smith, 1992). These monographs, valuable in themselves, do not attempt to place Medicare's range of conflicts into a broader portrait of American politics. Let me turn briefly to those that have tried to do so.

Two general books on American politics and medical care policy deserve special mention in that regard. Rushevsky and Patel's analysis of federal health policymaking in the 1990s portrays the institutional context in which Medicare's political fate in that decade was decided. (Rushevsky and Patel, 1998). The same is true for the broad study by Carol and William Weissert, who survey the scholarship on American politics generally and try to show how that illuminates the fate not only of Medicare but also of a variety of federal health programs (Weissert and Weissert, 1996).

Illuminating in a quite different way is Jacob Hacker's book on the fate of the Clinton health reform effort (Hacker 1997). *The Road to Nowhere* explains better than any other analysis why President Clinton selected the "managed competition" strategy for his "comprehensive" reform plan. Hacker's analysis of the role of competitive conceptions of health reform is crucial for understanding how those ideas resurfaced in 1995 in Republican Medicare proposals and migrated over time to a wider audience, culminating during 1999 in the Breaux-Thomas legislative proposal. I have relied to a considerable extent on Hacker's work for my understanding of the growth of pro-competitive conceptions of health reform since the 1970s.

Analysts of Medicare's politics have been hampered to date by the lack of a comprehensive history of the program's politics. Not surprisingly, the journal literature on Medicare's post-enactment politics has also been somewhat limited. One seminal article by Larry Brown was published in the mid-1980s (Brown, 1985). The same dating applies to Morone and Dunham's prescient article on how America slouches rather than moves decisively towards national health insurance (Morone and Dunham, 1985). Most analyses of Medicare's post-enactment politics have focused more on disputes about Medicare's regulatory policies than on the program's benefits and financing. The major exception is Himelfarb's book on the passage and repeal of the Medicare catastrophic protection bill in the late 1980s (Himelfarb, 1995).

Noting the relatively limited amount of scholarly writing on Medicare's politics highlights a general feature of Medicare commentary: namely, the high proportion of the considerable research on Medicare's operation that sets aside its politics entirely or incorporates presumptions about politics into the background. Another way of putting the same point is to say that most health services research and writing reveals one of two scholarly features (or "sins" to some). The bulk of such work either omits Medicare's politics altogether in analyses of programmatic developments or proposed reforms, or characterizes those politics with largely unexamined and undefended presumptions (Oberlander, 1995). Both forms shape understanding of this central program of American social policy.

Marilyn Moon's *Medicare: Now and In the Future* (Moon, 1993 and 1996) is a noteworthy illustration of the first category: a highly competent survey of the Medicare program on which I have very much relied. It is a work whose reluctance to discuss Medicare's politics is in some respects as illuminating as its detailed program portraiture. Moon begins by noting that Medicare, though a "fascinating and complex healthcare program", is "often not well understood" (Moon, 1993, xv). Her aim was to improve that understanding by providing the "overview" of Medicare's post-1965 development that, she rightly claimed, has been missing from the literature.

Moon does set the record straight on a number of matters. She gives a clear description of the growth of the Medicare program, noting its expansion after 1972 from an elderly constituency to one including not only the disabled, but also those of any age with renal failure. Moon provides accurate data on Medicare's outlays over time, rightly attacking two misconceptions that bedevil intelligent debate about the program's future. First, she notes that Medicare's annual rate of increase in per capita expenditures fell below the average national rate for private health insurance after 1985 after two decades of more rapid growth. Second, Moon debunks the notion that the aging of America's population, "must be a major factor in Medicare's growth." The number of beneficiaries is rising at only about 1.1 percent per year, hardly enough to account for much of Medicare's cost explosion since enactment. And this is but one of the myths Moon's financial and demographic account provides.

Medicare Now and in the Future distinctively and rightly emphasizes problems with the program that are clear to participants, but opaque to the public. One is the persistent increase after the program's start in the cost-sharing borne by Medicare's beneficiaries. Medicare began with benefits modeled after conventional Blue Cross/Blue Shield programs of the postwar period. Deductibles and coinsurance provisions were unthinkingly assumed to be necessary to keep the program's costs within reasonable bounds. But those features, when linked to the exclusion of most long-term care, loose control of what physicians could charge above the Medicare fee schedule, and the exclusion of payment for drugs, have meant that Medicare's beneficiaries pay on average very hefty sums. For example, "in 1986, elderly persons with a hospital stay and incomes of less than $10,000 spent 18.3 percent of their own income for acute health care services" (Moon, 1993, 11).

What Medicare spent, to whom and for whom, is where Moon's analysis is best. She treats marginal policy changes as needed, but deals very little with the political barriers to doing so. She reviews the difficulties with trying to reduce Medicare's costs substantially, but does not address the political barriers to doing so sensibly.

Marilyn Moon's approach is in many respects representative of how policy analysts in Washington deal with politics. There is a conventional way of presenting the analysis of policy, whether historical, contemporary, or prescriptive, a mode Allison describes as the "Unitary Actor Model" and featured in Chapter 5. This model presumes that one considers the country as a person, ask what problems there are with current behavior, and assume that a rational agent will in time review the options and choose sensible means to agreed-upon ends. Moon, like others in this craft tradition, knows this cannot be descriptively accurate. But, with the exception of her case study of catastrophic health insurance in the 1980s, Moon fails to incorporate political analysis into her account. In part, this posture reflects the division of intellectual labor between political and policy analysts. In part, it also illustrates that policy analysts present their views within the context of accepted notions of what politics permits.

The result is unrealistic—both in the "overview" of how the program developed and in what the future portends. Her bibliography is strikingly innocent of the work of political and social analysts like Larry Brown of Columbia, Theda Skocpol of Harvard, Jim Morone of Brown, Tom Oliver of Maryland, and Larry Jacobs of Minnesota. (I note exceptions here; Paul Starr's *The Social Transformation of American Medicine* and my book, *The Politics of Medicare* are cited, but hardly anything else I or other sociologists and political scientists have written over the past quarter century.) The most generous view of this is that the division of labor has benefits and Moon is an economist. The less generous view is that, for the understanding of public programs, a political economy approach is a necessary, if not sufficient condition of producing real illumination (Marmor, 1995).

There is another form of Medicare commentary in which political contentions are presented as self-evident even when they are contestable.

Consider, for illustrative purposes, the claim by Brookings' economists Henry Aaron and Robert Reischauer that "[f]ive central facts will shape the debate on the future of Medicare" (1995). According to Aaron and Reischauer:

> First, Medicare enjoys overwhelming support among the American electorate, a popularity that is well deserved because the program has achieved all of its designers' major objectives. Second, the cost of providing Medicare benefits is projected to rise very rapidly and will exceed projected revenues by ever larger amounts. Third, legislative reform of the entire health care system is now off the political agenda and likely will remain so for years to come. Fourth, there exists a strong and broad consensus against raising taxes. Fifth, dramatic changes are taking place in the way health care is financed and delivered for the non-Medicare population.
>
> The implications of these facts are straightforward. First, before changes are made in Medicare, policymakers will have to assure the general population and beneficiaries alike that the reforms will not compromise the attributes of the program that the public values so much. Second, Congress will have to act soon to restore Medicare's financial viability. Third, the measures that Congress adopts will not be part of any major legislative effort to reform the overall health care system. Fourth, most, if not all, of the budgetary savings on Medicare will come from reducing federal payments to providers and raising costs to beneficiaries, not from raising Medicare payroll taxes. Fifth, congressional reforms will—and should—bring Medicare more in line with the structure of health care financing and delivery that is evolving to serve the non-Medicare population (4–5).

As Jon Oberlander and I have noted elsewhere, these claims are mixtures of plausible surmises with historical inaccuracy, possible scenarios presented as certain fact, facts set out as if they were open to only one interpretation, and forecasts of the distant future that are not rooted in the indeterminacy of political and economic predictions (Marmor and Oberlander, 1998). Let me simply take one claim—the assertion that congressional reforms "will (and should) bring Medicare more in line with the structure of health care financing and delivery that is evolving to serve the non-Medicare population"—where the grounds for objection are obvious.

Note three features of this claim. There is first the conflation of predictive and normative judgement. It is clear that both are important types of judgement, but they lose credibility when casually conjoined. Second, there is the recommendation that Medicare should be adapted to what itself is "evolving." This assumes but does not examine seriously the belief that Medicare must, as a practical matter of avoiding resentment, resemble the health insurance practices affecting other Americans. Nor does the claim rest on any demonstrated superiority of the "evolving" practices. Instead, as I learned in a later exchange, (Marmor and Oberlander, 1998), Aaron and Reischauer are certain that Americans will increasingly resent Medicare beneficiaries who have more choice of provider than they do. There is no credible evidence to support this claim and what evidence there is suggests just the opposite.

Another issue raised by politically presumptive writing concerns predictions about the political agenda over time. The commentary on Medicare, as with other programs, is regularly accompanied by claims about what the future will be like years and decades into the future. My contention about confident futurology, presented elsewhere, is that configurations of partisan balance and economic circumstances cannot be easily anticipated and that considerable humility, for political scientists as well, is warranted (Marmor, 1999).

One of the most striking features of Medicare's political evolution is how the ideological cleavage that attended its birth reappeared, in a different guise, more than three decades later. Most reform advocates, for obvious reasons, claim an interest in "saving Medicare." But the equally obvious truth is that the program still excites fundamental differences about the proper role of government in health insurance. For those who embrace its social insurance purposes, this would be satisfaction. For those who reject those principles as inappropriate, the fight over "reforming" Medicare is in fact about changing it fundamentally. For an interesting and illuminating discussion of these matters, see the 1999 reports of the National Academy of Social Insurance Task Force on Medicare, especially the one on "Medicare's Social Role" (National Academy of Social Insurance, 1999).

In writing the chapters of Part II, I have relied much more on the secondary literature than was the case with the first edition of this book. At the same time, my understanding of the political environment facing Medicare came from broader research and writing projects that did not have the politics of the program as its central focus. My understandings of the context of American social welfare politics in the period 1966–90 are set out most explicitly in a coauthored work (Marmor, Mashaw and Harvey, 1992). My views about American medical care politics in this period are most fully discussed in a book of essays on *Understanding Health Care Reform* (Marmor, 1994). Finally, I want to acknowledge earlier versions of these chapters. An earlier version of Chapter 7 was published in *American Journal of Philosophy and Medicine* and again in Marmor and Mashaw, *Social Security: Beyond the Rhetoric of Crisis* (Marmor and Mashaw, 1998). And an earlier version of Medicare's relationship to the Clinton health reform effort appeared in *The American Prospect* (Marmor, 1993).

Glossary

Acute Care: Medical care of limited duration for an injury or short-term illness. A physician usually but not always provides such care in an office, clinic, or hospital.

Administrative Costs: Expenditures for delivering and managing the nonmedical aspects of care (for example, billing, claims processing, marketing, and overhead). Included are (a) the direct costs of insurance managers; (b) the indirect costs paid by other providers for such activities; (c) the nonmonetary costs to patients of dealing with insurance eligibility and billing.

Adverse Selection: The process whereby individuals who know they are most at risk of needing to file an insurance claim disproportionately purchase insurance and increase the costs of the insurance pool.

Aid to Families with Dependent Children (AFDC): A joint federal-state program (sometimes called welfare) that provides grants to those low-income individuals and their dependent children who meet eligibility requirements.

Alliance for Health Reform (AHR): A nonprofit organization that coordinated conferences and distributes information regarding health care reform; founded in 1991 by Senator John D. Rockefeller IV (D., W.Va.).

Alliance for Managed Competition: A lobbying organization formed by the major health insurance companies in the early 1990s.

All-Payer System: A system of reimbursement under which government and private insurance plans ("all payers") pay the same amount for the same service. For instance, federal-state **Medicaid** insurance programs would not be able to reimburse hospitals at a lower rate than a private insurer such as **Blue Cross**. The health provider thus could not shift costs from one payer to another.

Ambulatory Care: Services provided to individuals who are not inpatients in a medical institution.

American Association of Retired Persons (AARP): A lobbying group for individuals aged 50 or older. Founded in 1958, it has approximately 33 million members as of the late 1990s.

American Health Security Act: The name of the legislation that President Clinton proposed to Congress in 1993 to "reform" the provision and financing of U.S. medical care.

American Hospital Association (AHA): A trade association representing hospitals, health care facilities, and medical administrators. Founded in 1898, it has 50,000 members, about a tenth of which are hospitals.

American Medical Association (AMA): An organization founded in 1847 that as of 1999 represented 296,000 of this country's 600,000 doctors.

Bad Debt and Free Care: Both terms apply to hospital bills that are not paid. Free care technically refers to the expenses of those too poor to be expected to pay. Bad debt usually (but not always) refers to bills left unpaid by those who reasonably might be expected to pay.

Benefits: See Health Benefits.

Blue Cross/Blue Shield Association: The nonprofit national organization of 69 independent corporations that constitutes the oldest and largest private health insurer in the United States and the largest third-party administrator of **Medicare** benefits. Its affiliates provide health insurance to more than 67.5 million Americans.

Canadian Plan: The national health insurance system—administered by the 10 provinces—that covers the hospital care, outpatient care, and some prescription drugs for all Canadians. Usually called a **Single-Payer System**, Canada's "Medicare" is financed 38 percent by national taxation and 62 percent by provincial taxation. Private doctors in **Fee-for-Service** practices bill the provincial health ministries monthly; community-owned hospitals negotiate annual budgets with the provincial governments. The provincial governments set rates limiting the fees that providers can charge.

Capitation: A payment method in which a doctor or hospital is paid a fixed amount per patient per year—regardless of the services used by the patient. The method is used by some American HMOs, but is a form of reimbursement found in many organizational settings. It is the way most British and Dutch general practitioners are paid.

Case Management: One way of handling patients in **Managed Care** systems; also known as gatekeeping. In **Primary-Care** case management, a practitioner determines how much and what kinds of service (including that of specialists) a patient requires. **Acute-Care** case management usually deals with high- cost, seriously ill patients; a case manager monitors services and can arrange for alternative treatments. The system is sometimes regarded as meddlesome, sometimes as helpful.

Catastrophic Coverage: Insurance that pays for very large health care expenses (usually associated with accidents or chronic illnesses and diseases, such as cancer and AIDS). In general, this coverage is expensive and hard to find.

Charity Care: Free health care given by doctors, nurses, and hospitals. (In 1956, the Internal Revenue Service mandated charity care for nonprofit hospitals, to keep their tax-exempt status; that ruling was rescinded in 1969 but many hospitals continue to provide free care.)

COBRA: The Consolidated Omnibus Budget Reconciliation Act of 1985. It requires employers to make it possible for individuals who lose their health insurance for various reasons to continue to purchase such coverage for two years with their own funds, through the employer's plan.

Coinsurance: The percentage of medical costs, not covered by insurance, that an individual must pay. (Many plans pay only 80 percent of hospital and doctor's costs.)

Community Rating: A method for determining the price of health insurance premiums (the yearly amount that individuals pay for coverage). A community rating premium is based on the average medical cost for all covered people in a geographic area. The system is historically associated with nonprofit **Blue Cross/Blue Shield** plans. Most of these plans abandoned community rating when forced to compete with commercial insurers in the 1950s and thereafter.

Continuum of Care: A range of services and care settings that patients may require at different stages of their illness.

Copayment: The flat fee that must be paid by patients when they use health care—despite their insurance. Such "copays" range from nominal fees per visit (say, three dollars at an HMO) to higher preset limits.

Cost Sharing: A provision of a health care plan that requires individuals to cover some part of their medical expenses. It may help to hold down costs by deterring individuals from seeking unnecessary care, or it may discourage necessary care. In universal insurance plans, cost sharing can be regarded as taxation on being sick and using services. Typical forms include **Deductibles, Copayment,** and **Coinsurance.**

Death Spiral: The term applied when **Adverse Selection** gets out of control and sets off successive waves of rate increases. At each stage, the healthier subscribers drop their insurance because it has become too expensive—and only those who know they will need it (those who are sick) retain coverage.

Deductible: The amount a patient must pay out of pocket before health insurance will finance subsequent costs. (See **Cost Sharing**)

Defensive Medicine: Performing or ordering tests or procedures that would not have otherwise been performed, in order to be able to defend against a potential **Malpractice** claim.

Diagnosis-Related Groups (DRGs): A classification system adopted by **Medicare** in 1983 to set standard Medicare payments for hospitalization. Payments are predetermined based on the patient's diagnosis, having been adjusted for the average cost of such care in the area. After physicians determine the relevant diagnosis, Medicare reimburses the hospital regardless of the particular costs of the beneficiary's hospitalization.

Direct Employer Coverage: Health insurance obtained through an individual's employer (current or former), union, or family member. (Sixty percent of Americans are insured through their own employer or that of a family member.)

Employee Retirement Income Security Act (ERISA): A 1974 federal law that set the standards of disclosure for employee benefit plans, to ensure workers the right to at least part of their pension. The law governs most private pensions and other employee benefits, and overrides all state laws that concern employee benefits, including **Health Benefits.** The result has been the exclusion from state insurance regulations of the self-insured health plans of many large companies.

Employer Mandate: A requirement that all employers offer and nominally pay for a portion (in the Clinton plan, 80 percent) of their workers' health coverage. Many small businesses seem to fear that a health insurance mandate would be so costly that it would drive them out of business. Most analysts believe that the costs of employer mandates are largely borne by employees.

Entitlements: Government benefits, including health insurance, that are conferred automatically to all eligible individuals. They are part of mandatory spending programs such as Social Security, **Medicare**, **Medicaid**, and food stamps. The first two of these programs have a contributory taxation form of finance that underlies the concept of entitlement; the latter two do not.

ESRD: A funding program under **Medicare** for end-stage renal disease that pays for kidney dialysis and kidney transplants, enacted in 1972.

Experience Rating: A method used to determine the price of health insurance premiums based on the amount a certain group (such as the employees of a business) has previously paid for medical services. Indemnity insurance companies most often use experience rating when determining premium rates. Small businesses, however, can be hurt by experience rating, because one employee's severe medical problems can cause a significant increase in the entire group's premiums.

Fee for Service: A method of reimbursement where payment is made for a specific service. That fee can be fixed (a fee schedule) or derived from more complicated data (relative value scales).

First Party: The patient, in insurance lingo.

Formularies: Lists of approved drugs, which are the only ones that can be prescribed by physicians participating in certain programs. The list generally excludes more expensive options when cheaper, equally effective drugs are available.

Generic Drugs: Drugs essentially identical to brand-name versions without the brand name and without the higher price of the original product.

Global Budget: An amount, set by an administrative body, that controls the funds available to pay for medical care services in a region, state, or nation. Usually covering government spending and other insurance payers, global budgets are most often associated with universal health insurance, under which all individuals in a country are covered.

Group Health Association: A trade association made up of the major HMOs.

Health Benefits: Payments made by a health insurance firm to patients or medical providers to cover all or some of the costs of medical care.

Health Care Financing Administration (HCFA): Part of the Department of Health and Human Services, HCFA administers **Medicare** and **Medicaid**; it also records Medicare, Medicaid, and national health statistics. Created in 1977.

Health Industry Manufacturers' Association (HIMA): A trade association composed of manufacturers of medical devices, diagnostic products, and health care information systems, founded in 1974.

Health Insurance Association of America (HIAA): This organization, founded in 1956, represents 270 health insurance firms that write and sell individual and group policies.

Health Maintenance Organization (HMO): A prepaid medical care plan in which the organization receives a certain amount (usually monthly), and patients seek treatment from its affiliated medical staff. The goal is to provide affordable health care through organizational forms often called **Managed Care**—in which a **Primary-Care** provider is supposed to act as gatekeeper to specialists and expensive medical tests. Often subscribers pay a small amount at each visit. Patients in HMOs have variable limits on their choice of doctors.

Staff model.   Doctors are salaried and work only for the HMO, often at a single site.

Group model.   Doctors are organized in an independent partnership, corporation, or association that contracts only with the HMO.

Network model.   Combines two or more types of HMOs.

Health Plans: A phrase that has several meanings: (1) the networks of doctors, hospitals, and insurers that would, in the Clinton proposal, provide coverage through contracts negotiated with regional or corporate **Health Alliances**; (2) the benefits offered by health insurance providers to individuals and companies; (3) methods of paying for health care.

Holdbacks: Sums of money due to doctors in an HMO or other **Managed-Care** system that are not paid until overall volume for the period can be determined. If volume proves to be higher than planned, enough funds are permanently withheld to meet preset expenditure targets.

Indemnity Insurance: A form of health insurance in which the patient submits the medical bill to the insurance company for a specified level of reimbursement, which may be equal to or less than the fee charged.

Independent Practice Association (IPA): A form of medical practice in which physicians can treat both HMO and private patients. The HMO patients are charged a negotiated rate, usually on a per capita or fixed fee-for-service basis.

Indirect Employer Coverage: Insurance provided by an employer to the employees' family members, who may or may not receive fewer benefits than the employees.

Integrated Service Network (ISN): A new type of medical plan— one that offers broad medical care coverage—being developed in Minnesota. Quasi-public cooperatives and the state **Medicaid** system will negotiate rates and terms with the networks on behalf of large groups of consumers.

Jackson Hole Group: An informal group of business figures and academics who have met for some years at the Jackson Hole, Wyoming, home of Dr. Paul Ellwood to promote their preferred form of health care policy. (Ellwood previously worked for Inter-Study, a Minnesota health policy research company.) The group devised the Jackson Hole plan.

"Job Lock": Workers remain in a job for fear of losing health insurance coverage altogether, or because a prospective employer's health plan refuses to cover a medical circumstance such as a dependent's **Preexisting Condition**.

Long-Term Care: Health care required by chronically ill, physically disabled, or mentally disabled individuals. Such patients usually require round-the-clock supervision in a hospital, nursing home, or (less frequently) at home.

Loss Experience: The amount health insurance companies pay for the health care their policyholders use.

Major Medical: Refers usually to health insurance policies designed to cover substantial expenses associated with serious illness. Typically, policyholders pay extremely high deductibles— $25,000 per year, for example—before coverage starts and may pay **Coinsurance** of 20 percent as well.

Malpractice: Harmful treatment or neglect of a patient by a doctor or other medical provider, which is deemed professionally unacceptable.

Managed Care: An expression that means different things to different people. Sometimes it refers to efforts to control costs by using gate keepers—**Primary-Care** doctors or caseworkers—to coordinate the use of medical services by patients. Other times, it refers to networks organized by insurance companies, employers, or hospitals. An example is the type of network run by HMOs, in which a patient sees one doctor, who determines the medical care, both general and specialized, that he or she will receive. The patient's access to medical services is thereby controlled.

Managed Competition: Both a slogan and a set of ideas about health care reform. Largely embraced by President Clinton as an early label for his reform proposal, it proved a complicated marketing term and was abandoned as a Clinton policy tag. The concept of managed competition combines market forces with government regulation. Large groups of consumers buy medical care (or insurance for care) from networks of providers. The aim is to create price competition among those networks and thereby both restrain prices and encourage high-quality care and responsiveness. The variation among plans described as managed competition is substantial. The label is accordingly of uncertain worth.

Medicaid: The federal-state health insurance program for the categorically poor. Enacted in 1965, Medicaid took effect the following year. While program details differ from state to state, all states together spent $50 billion on Medicaid in 1992, and the federal government spent $68 billion. In that year Medicaid paid for the care of 32.6 million people, spending nearly a third of its budget on **Long-Term Care**.

Medicaid Waiver: The formal process by which a state receives federal permission to deviate from certain **Medicaid** program rules. The most controversial U.S. example of this process involved the State of Oregon's plan to widen Medicaid eligibility while narrowing (**Rationing**) the range of services it said it would finance.

Medical Savings Accounts: Analogous to individual retirement accounts, but employers and employees can make tax-deferred contributions and employees can withdraw funds to pay covered medical expenses.

Medicare: The federal health insurance program for the elderly and disabled enacted in 1965 and started a year later. Its benefits include hospital care, doctor visits, and other services. Financed by individual premiums, social insurance taxes, and general revenues, Medicare is the largest federal health program today, covering not only the elderly but also the disabled and those with chronic renal failure. Largely omitted from the Clinton reform proposal, Medicare expansion was the basis of other proposals—most prominently that of Congressman Fortney (Pete) Stark (D., Calif.).

Part A. The Medicare program that pays for hospital care. As of 1992 it covers inpatient care beyond a $676 deductible and also provides short-term nursing care. Medicare Part A cost $80.8 billion that year and covered 34.4 million people. It is financed by a 1.15 percent payroll tax.

Part B. The so-called voluntary part of Medicare, known as Supplementary Medical Insurance, which pays a portion of doctors' bills. Medicare Part B is supposed to pay 80 percent of a physician's fee, once the beneficiary has met a $100 deductible. Covering 33.6 million people in 1992, Medicare Part B expenditures were $48.6 billion. The program is financed by patient premiums and general federal revenues in a ratio of roughly one to four.

Medicare Catastrophic Coverage Act: Passed by Congress in 1988, this law provided benefits for those with catastrophic medical problems, capped out-of-pocket expenses, and covered prescription drugs. But after many senior citizens objected to the new program's financing and rationale, Congress repealed the law in 1989.

Medicare + Choice: The option for Medicare beneficiaries legislated in the Balanced Budget Act of 1997. The Plus Choice element widened the alternatives to Medicare's traditional service benefits; the additional enrollment possibilities included medical savings accounts, preferred provider organizations (PPSs), provider sponsored organizations (PSOs), and private fee-for-service plans. For such options, Medicare beneficiaries continue to pay Part B premiums, but must get all Medicare-covered benefits through the private plan chosen.

Medigap: Private health insurance plans that augment **Medicare** by paying medical bills not covered by the federal government. Payments could include **Coinsurance**, coverage of Medicare **Deductibles**, and bills not covered by Medicare (including prescription drugs).

National Health Budget: The total amount spent on health care by government and private payers. In 1992 the United States spent

$832 billion—one-seventh of the entire U.S. economic output. The Congressional Budget Office estimates that the cost may rise to $1.6 trillion by the year 2000.

National Health Care: A misleading label for a health insurance system that covers all citizens and various other residents. Sometimes it is the designation for so-called **Single-Payer** version of national health insurance, particularly those modeled after Canada's system. Under such a plan, the government sets all budgets for hospitals and fees for doctors and other providers.

Oregon Plan: See **Rationing**.

Per-Person Premium: A flat-rate health insurance premium, as opposed to a premium for a family or one based on a percentage of income.

Pharmaceutical Manufacturers' Association (PMA): A trade association founded in 1958 that represents 88 companies within the industry that develop and manufacture prescription drugs.

Physician Payment Review Commission (PPRC): Recommends reimbursement rates for doctors in the **Medicare** program. Founded by Congress in 1986, the 13-member commission is charged with analyzing Medicare payment issues and submitting its findings to Congress. Congress then decides on the policies to be used, and HCFA sets the actual rate.

Play or Pay: A health insurance reform plan in which employers either provide their workers with a basic **Health Benefits** package ("play") or pay into a government insurance pool. The system was popular in 1991 among congressional Democrats.

Point-of-Service Plan (POS): A feature of a health insurance plan whereby patients are financially rewarded for using a limited group of providers, but are permitted to seek out-of-network care at higher cost.

Preexisting Condition: A physical or mental condition diagnosed before an individual receives health insurance coverage. Some insurers refuse to cover a person with such a condition; others increase their rates or refuse to cover the patient for a specific time. Preexisting conditions are the object of intense reform attention in 1994 as an example of how conventional insurance practices have hurt precisely those who need insurance most.

Preferred Provider Organization (PPO): Under this system providers, usually organized by networks or panels, offer medical care for a set fee. Various benefits, such as lower **Coinsurance** and better coverage, create incentives for patients to see "preferred" doctors; restrictions on caregivers are, by contrast, the disincentives.

Premium Tax: A state tax on the payments made to an insurance company by policyholders who live in that state.

Price Controls: Government-set price ceilings on goods or services. In medical care, the term usually refers to a physician fee schedule.

Primary Care: The care people routinely receive when they go to the doctor. Primary care can be delivered by a doctor, nurse practitioner, or physician's assistant. Doctors practicing family medicine, pediatrics, or internal medicine are generally considered primary-care providers.

Prior Approval: A form of utilization review whereby an insurance company requires a hospital or doctor to get permission from the insurance company before providing care.

Protocol: A guide for the treatment of a specific disease or condition.

Qualified Medicare Beneficiary: A person aged 65 or older whose income falls below the federal poverty line and for whom the **Medicaid** program must pay all Medicare costs, including Part B premiums, **Deductibles**, and **Copayments**.

Rate Setting: Refers generally to a government's setting of prices—whether for electricity, water, or health care. Maryland has had such a system for hospitals since the 1970s.

Rationing: Any process that in medical care limits the services a person can receive. Allocation based on income is widespread in the United States, as are other limits. Rationing is unavoidable in medical care, although the bases of rationing are varied and differently valued.

Reinsurance: See **Stop-Loss Coverage**.

Relative Value Scale (RVS): A method of establishing differential fees for physicians' services. The RVS was a 1992 effort by **Medicare** to shift funding away from **Specialists**, who were receiving relatively high Medicare payments, toward **Primary-Care** practitioners. It bases the value of each medical procedure on its complexity. The conversion factor chosen translates the number into a specific dollar amount.

Risk-Control Insurance: See **Stop-Loss Coverage**.

Risk Pool: A group of people brought together for purposes of pricing insurance. Sometimes the term refers to those who seek insurance but cannot, because of their medical history, get it (a "high"-risk pool). In the Clinton plan the risk pool consists of everyone within a **Health Alliance** or a **Health Plan**.

Second Party: The caregiver or provider. See also **Third-Party Payer**.

Self-Insurance: A form of health insurance in which an employer (or others)—but not an insurance company—assumes the risk of health expenses. Third parties may administer such plans.

Single-Payer Option: A provision of the Clinton plan that permitted a state to choose to make direct payments to medical providers, with no intermediaries.

Single-Payer System: A **Universal Coverage** plan under which the government collects funds for health insurance and has a uniform plan for everyone in a given state or nation. Canada has this form of universal health insurance administered in its ten provinces. The arrangements effectively eliminate private health insurance for basic coverage. Proponents claim it is the best way to control the rise in national health costs.

Specialist: Any physician who has pursued specialty training beyond the first year of residency. Often the term implies that the doctor does not provide **Primary Care**.

Spend Down: A requirement of many state **Medicaid** programs that individuals use up their assets when these are above the level required for eligibility to collect benefits.

Stop-Loss Coverage: Insurance by one insurer of all or part of a risk previously assumed by another insurer (or **Health Plan**). It is a form of backup insurance that reimburses a health plan (stops its losses) when the payments it makes exceed the expected outlays. Stop-loss coverage is also known as reinsurance or risk-control insurance.

Task Force on National Health Care Reform: The presidential advisory group, formed in January 1993 and chaired by Hillary Rodham Clinton, that worked for four months on a proposed overhaul of the American health insurance system. The task force comprised more than 500 people, largely technical specialists, drawn from within government and private organizations.

Third-Party Administrator: A person or corporate entity that handles the administrative details of health insurance for a **Self-Insured** group. The group assumes the financial risks: the third party does not.

Third-Party Payer: A person or organization that pays all or part of a set of medical expenses—but not the patient (the first party) or the caregiver (the second party). Examples are **Medicaid, Medicare, Blue Cross/Blue Shield**, and most commercial health insurance companies. A traditional HMO need not involve a third-party payer.

Uncompensated Care: Services given by hospitals or other providers not paid for by patients, their insurance companies, or the government. The cost of such care is often shifted to paying patients or their insurers.

Underinsured: Those persons—estimated at 15 million to 30 million in the United States—with inadequate health insurance. High **Deductibles**, limited coverage, unavailable providers, and waiting periods are all sources of inadequate coverage.

Uninsured: Those people without health insurance, estimated in 1991 at 36.6 million Americans with more than 40 million in 1999.

Universal Coverage: Refers to a situation where all (citizens-residents) have health insurance.

Utilization Review: A process by which an insurance company reviews decisions of doctors and hospitals on what care to provide for patients.

Volume Performance Standards: The number of physician services that the managers of a **Health Plan** expect to be provided in a given period.

Voucher: A grant of money for a restricted purpose, for example, a meal voucher. In connection with **Medicare**, the idea arose in 1995 as a way to limit the federal government's responsibility for financing the program. Then the conception was of a fixed sum available only to purchase health insurance with a minimum set of benefits. In 1999, the idea changed to a variable amount available to Medicare beneficiaries to be used in connection with what was a form of **Managed Competition**. The technical term for this variable voucher, in 1999, was "premium support," as in the Breaux-Thomas proposal.

Wage-Based Premium: Similar to a tax. this method of raising funds for health care requires all employers to pay a percentage of their payroll for their employees' health insurance. A small portion of the premium may be paid by the employee.

Workers' Compensation Insurance: Insurance that reimburses employers for the costs of compensating employees who are injured in the course of their employment.

References to Part I

Anderson, Odin (1968). *The Uneasy Equilibrium.* New Haven, CT: College & University Press.

Bauer, Raymond, A. Ithiel de Sola Pool, and Lewis Dexter (1963). *American Business and Public Policy.* New York: Atherton.

Burrow, James G. (1963). *AMA: Voice of American Medicine.* Baltimore: Johns Hopkins University Press.

Cantril, Hadley (1952). *Public Opinion: 1935–1946.* Princeton, NJ: Princeton University Press.

Cornwell, Elmer E., Jr. (1965). *Presidential Leadership of Public Opinion.* Bloomington: Indiana University Press.

Davis, Michael M. (1941). *America Organizes Medicine.* New York: Harper & Brothers.

Edelman, Murray (1964). *The Symbolic Uses of Politics.* Urbana: Illinois University Press.

Eidenberg, Eugene and Roy D. Morey (1969). *An Act of Congress.* New York: W. W. Norton.

Feingold, Eugene (1966). *Medicare: Policy and Politics.* San Francisco: Chandler.

Friedman, Lawrence (1968). *Government and Slum Housing.* Chicago: Rand McNally.

Greenfield, Margaret (1966). *Health Insurance for the Aged: The 1965 Program for Medicare.* Berkeley: Institute of Governmental Studies, University of California, 88, 26–28.

Hamilton, Richard F. (1972). *Class and Politics in the United States.* Chapter 2. New York: Wiley.

Harris, Richard (1966). *A Sacred Trust.* New York: New American Library.

Kelley, Stanley, Jr. (1966). *Professional Public Relations and Political Power.* Baltimore: Johns Hopkins University Press.

Key, V. 0. (1961). *Public Opinion and American Democracy.* New York: Knopf.

Meranto, Philip (1967). *The Politics of Federal Aid to Education in 1965.* Syracuse, NY: Syracuse University Press.

Mitchell, Joyce M. and William C. Mitchell (1969). *Political Analysis and Public Policy*. Chicago: Rand Mcnally, 162.

Munger, Frank J. and Richard F. Fenno (1962). *National Politics and Federal Aid to Education*. Syracuse, NY: Syracuse University Press.

Munts, Raymond (1967). *Bargaining for Health: Labor Unions, Health Insurance and Medical Care*. Madison: University of Wisconsin Press.

Peters, Clarence A., Ed. (1964). *Free Medical Care*. New York: H. W. Wilson.

Ranney, Austin, Ed., (1968). *Political Science and Public Policy*. Chicago: Markham.

Rose, Arnold M. (1967). *The Power Structure*. New York: Oxford University Press.

Somers, Herman and Anne Somers (1961). *Doctors, Patients, and Health Insurance*. Garden City, NY: Anchor.

Somers, Herman and Anne Somers (1967). *Medicare and the Hospitals: Issues and Prospects*. Washington, DC: Brookings Institution.

Stevens, R. and R. Stevens (1974). *Welfare Medicine in America*. New York: Free Press.

Wildavsky, Aaron (1962). *Dixon-Yates: A Study in Power Politics*. New Haven, CT: Yale University Press.

Articles

Allison, Graham T. (1968). "Conceptual Models and the Cuban Missile Crisis." Paper Presented at the 1968 Annual Meeting of the American Political Science Association, Washington, D.C., September 2–7.

Ball, Robert M. (1964). "The American Social Security Program." *New England Journal of Medicine* 270(January 30):232–36.

Cohen, Wilbur J. (1960). "Health Insurance under Social Security." Reprinted from *American Journal of Nursing* 60(April):5.

Cohen, Wilbur J. and Robert M. Ball (1965). "Social Security Amendments of 1965: Summary and Legislative History." *Social Security Bulletin* (September):5.

Friedman, Lawrence (1969). "Social Welfare Legislation." *Stanford Law Review* 21(January):247.

Gallup, George (1965). "Majority Backs Medical Care of Aged Through Social Security." *Public Opinion News Service* (January 3).

Hyde, Wolff, et al. (1954). "AMA: Power, Purpose, and Politics in Organized Medicine." *Yale Law Journal* (May).

Lowi, Theodore (1964). "American Business, Public Policy, and Political Theory." *World Politics* 16.

Manley, John F. (1965). "The House Committee on Ways and Means: Conflict Management in a Congressional Committee." *American Political Science Review* 59(December):927–39.

Marmor, Theodore (1968). "Why Medicare Helped Raise Doctors' Fees." *Transaction* (September):4.

Mayer, Martin (1949). "The Dogged Retreat of the Doctors." *Harper's* (December):36.

Nation's Business (1962). Cited in American Medical Association (1963b): 52–53.

New Republic (1962). "Evaluation of Ways and Means Democrats, First Session, Key Votes—87th Congress" (October 27).

New Republic (1965). "New Deal H." 152(March 20). *New York Times* (1965). "Medicare's Progress." March 25.

Rice, Dorothy P. and Loucelle A. Horowitz (1968). "Medical Care Price Changes in Medicare's First Two Years." *Social Security Bulletin* (November).

Schecter, Mal (1968). "Emergency Medicare and Desegregation: A Special Report." *Hospital Practice* (July):14–19, 63–64.

American Medical Association Publications

AMA (1961). *A National Legislative Program for County Medical Societies: Operation Hometown* (Chicago: AMA).

AMA (1963). *The Case Against the King-Anderson Bill (H.R. 3920)*. Statement of the American Medical Association before the

Committee on Ways and Means, House of Representatives, 89th Congress (Chicago: AMA). AMA (1965). "Why Eldercare Offers Better Care Than Medicare." *AMA Journal* (March).

Congressional Hearings

U.S. Congress (1961a). *Health Services for the Aged under the Social Security Insurance System* (H.R. 4222). Hearings before the Committee on Ways and Means, House of Representatives, 87th Congress, 1st Session, July–August.

U.S. Congress (1961b). Testimony of Secretary Ribicoff, Health Services for the Aged under the Social Security Insurance System. Hearings before the Committee on Ways and Means, House of Representatives, 87th Congress, 1st Session, I (July–August).

U.S. Congress (1965). *Trends in Quantity and Quality of Health Insurance Coverage among the Aged*. Executive Hearings, Ways and Means Committee, House of Representatives, 89th Congress, 1st Session, 40–44.

Congressional Reports

Legislative Reference Service, Education and Public Welfare Division (1963). *The Federal Government: Role in Providing Medicare to the Citizens of the U.S.* Library of Congress. Washington, DC: U.S.

Government Printing Office. U.S. Congress (1963). *The Kerr-Mills Program, 1960–1963.*

Report of Subcommittee on Health of the Elderly, Special Committee on Aging, U.S. Senate, 88th Congress, 1st Session (October), 1–4.

U.S. Congress (1965a). *Social Security Amendments of 1965*. Report of the Committee on Ways and Means of H.R. 6675, 89th Congress, 1st Session, Report No. 213. Washington, DC: U.S. Government Printing Office.

U.S. Congress (1965b). Summary of Major Provisions of House of Representatives 6675, the Social Security Amendments of 1965 as Agreed to by the House, Senate Conference Committee, Committee on Ways and Means, 89th Congress, 1st Session (July 21).

Congressional Quarterly Service Publications

Congressional Quarterly (1965a). *Congress and the Nation: 1945–1964*. Washington, DC: Congressional Quarterly Service.
Congressional Quarterly (1965b). *Legislators and the Lobbyists*. Washington, DC: Congressional Quarterly Service.
Congressional Quarterly (1965c). Weekly Report, June 25.
Congressional Quarterly (1965d). Weekly Report, January 1.

HEW Publications

HEW (1959). *Health Manpower Source Book,* Public Health Service Publication No. 263, Sec. 9. Washington, DC: U.S. Government Printing Office.
HEW, Social Security Administration (1962). *The Health Care of the Aged*. Washington, DC: U.S. Government Printing Office (22–32).
HEW (1964). *Chart Book of Basic Health Economic Data,* Public Health Service Publication No. 3. Washington, DC: U.S. Government Printing Office.
HEW (1965a). *Background Book on Hospital Insurance for the Aged Through Social Security-H.R. 1*. Unpublished data, IX-b-6.
HEW (1965b). Hew Memorandum, Alanson W. Willcox, General Counsel to Wilbur J. Cohen, Assistant Secretary (May 21, 1965), Re: H.R. 6675-Douglas Amendment on Hospital Specialists.
HEW (1967a). *A Report to the President on Medical Care Prices*. Washington, DC: U.S. Government Printing Office.
HEW (1967b). "Current Data from the Medicare Program." *Health Insurance Statistics* (November 20).
HEW (1967c). *A Report to the President on Medical Care Prices*. Washington, DC: U.S. Government Printing Office.

Unpublished Sources

Askey, Vincent, M. D. (1961). "Aging, Medicine, and Kerr-Mills." Address delivered before the California Medical Association, Los Angeles, May 1.
Bray, Howard—Staff Member (1965). "Memorandum on Important Defects in H.R. 6675 Currently under Discussion in the Senate Finance Committee." (May 20).
Cohen, Wilbur J.—Assistant Secretary, HEW (1965). "Memorandum for the President," March 2.
Mills, Wilbur D. (1964). "Financing Health Care for the Aged." Address before Downtown Little Rock Lions Club, Little Rock, Arkansas (December 7).

Duplicated in HEW Background for the 1965 Legislative Session, IX-B-1, January 25.

Quealy, William H.—Minority Counsel (1965). "Memorandum to Ways and Means Republicans" (January 17).

Somers, Anne (1968). *Total Financing of Health Care: Past, Present, and Future.*

Vinyard, Dale (1972). "The Senate Committee on the Aging and the Development of a Policy System." Paper delivered at the Political Science Section of Michigan Academy, East Lansing, Michigan, March.

References to Part II

Aaron, H. J. and R. D. Reischauer (1995). "The Medicare ReformDebate: What Is the Next Step?" *Health Affairs* 14(Winter,11):8.

Aaron, H. J. and R. D. Reischauer (1998). "'Rethinking Medicare Reform' Needs Rethinking." *Health Affairs* 17(January/February, 1):69–71.

Allison, Graham T. and P.I. Zelikon (1999). *Essence of Decision: Explaining the Cuban Missile Crisis*. 2d ed. New York: Longman.

Americans for Generational Equity (1990). Annual Report. Washington, DC: Author.

Ball, R. M. (1972). Assignment of the Commissioner of Social Security. December 18 (unpublished report).

Ball, R. M. (1988). "The Original Understanding on Social Security: Implications for Later Developments." In T. R. Marmor and J. L. Mashaw (Eds.), *Social Security: Beyond the Rhetoric of Crisis* (pp. 17–40). Princeton, NJ: Princeton University Press.

Blendon, R. J., et al. (1990). "Satisfaction with Health Systems in Ten Nations." *Health Affairs* 9(2):185–92.

Bowler, M. K. (1987). "Changing Politics of Federal Health Insurance Programs." *PS* 20(2):202–11.

Brown, L. D. (1983). *Politics and Health Care Organization: HMOs as Federal Policy*. Washington, DC: Brookings Institution Press.

Brown, L. D. (1985). "Technocratic Corporatism and Administrative Reform in Medicare." *Journal of Health Politics, Policy and Law* 10(3):579–99.

Brown, L. D. (1996). "The Politics of Medicare and Health Reform, Then and Now." *Health Care Financing Review* 18(Winter, 2):163–68.

Butler, S. M. and E. F. Haislmaier (Eds.) (1989). *A National Health System for America*. Washington, DC. The Heritage Foundation.

Castellblanch, R. (1999). "Medicare's Critical Condition." *In These Times* (May 2):12–14.

Chicago Tribune (1995). "Democrats Use Umbrellas to Protest GOP Medicare Plans." September 22.

Christianson, J. B. and W. McClure (1979). "Competition in the Delivery of Medical Care." *New England Journal of Medicine* 301:812.

Concord Coalition (1992). *The Concord Coalition: Citizens for America's Future.* Washington, DC: Author.

Congressional Budget Office (1997). "January 1997 Baseline: Medicare." Washington, DC: Government Printing Office.

Conrad, D. and T. R. Marmor (1983). "Patient Cost Sharing." In Theodore R. Marmor (Ed.), *Political Analysis and American Medical Care Essays* (Chapter 11). New York: Cambridge University Press.

Corning, P. A. (1969). *The Evolution of Medicare . . . from Idea to Law.* Washington, DC: U.S. Government Printing Office.

David, S. I. (1985). *With Dignity: The Search for Medicare and Medicaid.* Westport, CT: Greenwood.

Daniels, Norman (1988). *Am I My Parents' Keeper: An Essay on Justice between the Young and the Old.* New York: Oxford University Press.

Davis, K. (1985). "Access to Health Care: A Matter of Fairness." In *Health Care: How to Improve It and Pay for It.* Washington, DC: Center for National Policy.

Demkovich, L. E. (1980). "Competition Coming On." *National Journal* 12: 1152.

Derthick, Martha, and Paul J. Quirk (1985). *The Politics of Deregulation.* Washington, DC: Brookings Institution.

Dionne, E. J. (1996). "Stealing Republican Issues." *New Statesman* (December 6).

Etheredge, L. (1997). "The Medicare Reforms of 1997: Headlines You Didn't Read." Paper presented at the American Political Science Association Meetings, Washington, DC, August 27.

Evans, R. G. (1986). "Finding the Levers, Finding the Courage: Lessons from Cost Containment in North America." Journal of Health Politics and Law 11(4):585–615.

Evans, R. G., et al. (1989). "Controlling Health Expenditures: The Canadian Reality." *New England Journal of Medicine* 320:572.

Evans, R. G., M. L. Barer, and C. Hertzman (1991). "The 20-Year Experiment: Accounting for, Explaining, and Evaluating Health Care Cost Containment in Canada and the United States." *Annual Review of Public Health* 12:481–518.

Evans, R. G., M. L. Barer, and G. L. Stoddart (1994). *Charging Peter to Pay Paul: Accounting for the Financial Effects of User Charges.* Toronto: Premier's Council on Health, Well-being and Social Justice.

Fallows, J. (1995). "A Triumph at Misinformation." *Atlantic Monthly* (January 26).

Feder, J. M. (1977). *Medicare: The Politics of Federal Hospital Insurance.* Lexington, MA: Lexington.

Feder, J. M., J. Holahan, and T. R. Marmor (Eds.) (1980). *National Health Insurance: Conflicting Goals and Policy Choices.* Washington, DC: Urban Institute Press.

Fox, D. M. (1986). *Health Policies, Health Politics: The British and American Experience, 1911–1965.* Princeton, NJ: Princeton University Press.

Freeland, M. S. and C. E. Schendler (1984). "Health Spending in the 1980's." *Health Care Financing Review* (Spring):1–68.

Fuchs, V. R. (1990). "The Health Sector's Share of the Gross National Product." *Science* 247:534–37.

Fuchs, V. R. and J. S. Hahn (1990). "How Does Canada Do It?" *New England Journal of Medicine* 323–386: 884–890.

Gallup, George (1991). Public Opinion Newsletter.

Gallup, George (1992). Public Opinion Newsletter.

Gallup, George (1993). Public Opinion Newsletter.

Gornick, M., et. al. (1985). "Twenty Years of Medicare and Medicaid: Covered Populations, Use of Benefits, and Program Expenditures." *Health Care Financing Review* (Annual Supplement):13–59.

Graetz, Michael J. and Jerry L. Mashaw (1999). *True Security.* New Haven, CT: Yale University Press.

Hacker, J. S. (1997). *The Road to Nowhere: The Genesis of President Clinton's Plan for Health Security.* Princeton, NJ: Princeton University Press.

Harris Poll (1999). #28, April 28. Lewis Harris and Associates, Inc. New York, New York.

Harvey, L. (1986). *AMA Surveys of Physician and Public Opinion: 1986.* Chicago: American Medical Association.

Herzlinger, R. (1991). "Healthy Competition." *Atlantic* 268:69–82.

Himelfarb, R. (1995). *Catastrophic Politics: The Rise and Fall of the Medicare Catastrophic Coverage Act of 1998.* University Park: Pennsylvania State University Press.

Himelfarb, R. (1997). "False Promises: Lessons from Recent Health Care Reform Catastrophes." Paper presented at the Midwest Political Science Association Meetings, Chicago, Illinois, April 10–12.

Himmelstein, D. U. and S. Woolhandler (1986). "Cost without Benefit: Administrative Waste in U.S. Health Care." *New England Journal of Medicine* 314:441–45.

House Committee on Ways and Means (1993). Hearing on President's Health Care Plan. October 21.

Jacobs, L. (1993). *Health of Nations.* Ithaca, NY: Cornell University Press.

Jacobs, L. (forthcoming). *Politicians Don't Pander: Political Manipulations and the Loss of Democratic Responses.* Chicago: University of Chicago Press.

Jacobs, L. R., R. Y. Shapiro, and E. Schulman (1993). "Poll Trends: Medical Care in the United States—An Update." *Public Opinion Quarterly,* 57(3): 394–427. Fall 1993.

Jost, T. (1999). "Governing Medicare." *Administrative Law Review* 51(1):40–116.

Kaiser Family Foundation (1999). "Voters Say Medicare Top Health Issue For New Congress." #1452. January 14.

Kuttner, Robert (1999). "Medicare Commission's Voucher Plan Is Bad News for Poor Elderly." Boston Globe, 17 January.

Letsch, Suzanne W., et al. (1992). "National Health Expenditures, 1991." *Health Care Financing Review* (Winter):1–30.

Light, P. (1986). *Artful Work: The Politics of Social Security Reform.* New York: Random House.

Lurie, N., et al. (1984). "Termination from Medi-Cal: Does It Affect Health?" *New England Journal of Medicine* 311(7):480–84.

Marmor, T. R. (1975). "Can the U.S. Learn from Canada?" In S. Andreopoulos (Ed.), *National Health Insurance: Can We Learn from Canada?* New York: Wiley.

Marmor, T. R. (1976). "The Politics of Medical Inflation. *Journal of Health Politics, Policy and Law* 1(1, Spring).

Marmor, T. R. (1987). "Entrepreneurship in Public Management." In J. Doig and E. Hargrove (Eds.), *Leadership and Innovation: A Biographical Perspective on Entrepreneurs in Government.* Baltimore, MD: Johns Hopkins University Press.

Marmor, T. R. (1988). "Coping with a Creeping Crisis: Medicare at Twenty." In T. R. Marmor and J. L. Mashaw (Eds.), *Social Security: Beyond the Rhetoric of Crisis.* Princeton, NJ: Princeton University Press.

Marmor, T. R. (1990). "American Health Politics, 1970 to the Present: Some Comments." *Quarterly Review of Economics and Business* 30(4):32–42.

Marmor, T. R. (1993). "Coalition or Collision? Medicare and Health Reform." *American Prospect* (Winter).

Marmor, T. R. (1994). *Understanding Health Care Reform.* New Haven, CT: Yale University Press.

Marmor, T. R. (1995). "Review of Marilyn Moon's 'Medicare: Now and In the Future.'" *Disability Studies Quarterly.*

Marmor, T. R. (1998a). "Forecasting American Health Care: How We Got Here and Where We Might Be Going." *Journal of Health Politics, Policy and Law* 23(3):551–71.

Marmor, T. R. (1998b). "Hope and Hyperbole: The Rhetoric and Reality of Managerial Reform in Health Care." *Journal of Health Services Research and Policy* 3(1, January).

Marmor, T.R. and J.B. Christianson (1982). *Health Care Policy: A Political Economy Approach.* Beverly Hills, CA: Sage Publications.

Marmor, T. R., R. Boyer, and J. Greenberg (1983). "Medical Care and Procompetitive Reform." In T. R. Marmor (Ed.), *Political Analysis and American Medical Care.* New York: Cambridge University Press.

Marmor, T. R. and J. S. Hacker (1997). "The Doomsayers Are Wrong." *Los Angeles Times*, July 24, B-9.

Marmor, T. R. and T. Hamburger (1993). "Dead on Arrival: Why Washington's Power Elites Won't Consider Single Payer Health Reform." *Washington Monthly* 25(September, 9):27–32.

Marmor, T. R., T. Hamburger, and J. Meacham (1994). "What the Death of Health Reform Teaches Us about the Press." *Washington Monthly* 26(11):35–41.

Marmor, T. R. and R. Klein (1986). "Cost vs. Care: America's Health Care Dilemma Wrongly Considered." *Health Matrix* 4(1, Spring).

Marmor, T. R. and J. L. Mashaw (Eds.) (1988). *Social Security: Beyond the Rhetoric of Crisis.* Princeton, NJ: Princeton University Press.

Marmor, T. R. and J. L. Mashaw (1996). "Can the American State Guarantee Access to Health Care?" In P. Fox, D. M. Fox, R. Maxwell, and E. Schrivan (Eds.), *The State, Politics and Health: Essays for Rudolf Klein.* Cambridge, MA: Blackwell.

Marmor, T. R., J. Mashaw, and P. Harvey (1990). "Crisis and the Welfare State." In T. Marmor, J. Mashaw and P. Harvey (Eds), *America's Misunderstood Welfare State: Persistent Myths, Enduring Realities.* New York: Basic Books.

Marmor, T. R. and J. A. Morone (1981). "Representing Consumer Interest: The Case of American Health." *Ethics* 91(April).

Marmor, T. R. and J. A. Morone (1983). "The Health Programs of the Kennedy-Johnson Years: An Overview." In T. R. Marmor (Ed.), *Political Analysis and Medical Care: Essays.* New York: Cambridge University Press.

Marmor, T. R. and J. B. Oberlander (1998). "Rethinking Medicare Reform." *Health Affairs* 17(1):52–58.

Marmor, T. R., M. Schlesinger, and R. W. Smithey (1986). "A New Look at Nonprofits: Health Care Policy in a Competitive Age." *Yale Journal on Regulation* 3(2):313–49.

Melhado, E. M. (1988). "Competition Versus Regulation in American Health Policy." In E. M. Melhado, W. Feinberg, and H. M. Swartz (Eds.), *Money, Power, and Health Care.* Ann Arbor, MI: Health Administration Press.

Mondale, W. (1978). "The Case for the Hospital Cost Containment Act." In *Controlling Health Care Costs.* Washington, DC: Government Research Corporation.

Moon, M. (1993). *Medicare Now and in the Future.* Washington, DC: Urban Institute Press.

Moon, M. (1996). *Medicare Now and in the Future* (2nd ed.). Washington, DC: Urban Institute Press.

Moon, M., and S. Zuckerman (1995). "Are Private Insurers Really Controlling Spending Better Than Medicare?" Henry Kaiser Family Foundation, July. Menlo Park, CA.

Morone, James A. and Andrew B. Dunham (1985). "Slouching towards National Health Insurance: The New Health Care Politics." *Yale Journal on Regulation* 2:263.

Morone, James A. (1994). "The Administration of Health Care Reform." *Journal of Health Politics, Policy and Law* 19 (1): 233-37.

National Academy of Social Insurance (1999). Final Report of the Study Panel on Medicare's Larger Social Role, "Medicare and the American Social Contract." February 1999. Washington, DC: Author.

National Academy on an Aging Society (1999). *Demography Is Not Destiny.* Washington, DC: Author.

New York Times (1998). "So Far, Medicare Plus Choice Is Minus Most of the Options." October 4, p. C10.

Oberlander, J. B. (1995). *Medicare and the American State.* Ph.D. dissertation, Yale University. Available from UMI Dissertation Service, Ann Arbor, Michigan.

Oberlander, J. B. (1997). "Managed Care and Medicare Reform." *Journal of Health Politics, Policy and Law* 22(2):595–631.

Oberlander, J. B. (1998). "Medicare: The End of Consensus." Paper Prepared for Presentation at the Annual Meetings of the American Political Science Association, Boston, September.

Oberlander, J. (1999). "Medicare: The End of Consensus." Paper presented at the annual meetings of the American Political Science Association, Boston, MA, September 1999.

Oliver, T. (1993). "Analysis, Advice, and Congressional Leadership: The Physician Payment Review Commission and the Politics of Medicare." *Journal of Health Politics, Policy and Law* 18(1):113–74.

Oliver, T. (1996). *Conceptualizing the Challenges of Public Sector Entrepreneurship.* Westport, CT: Praeger.

Patashnik, E. M. (2000). *Putting Trust in the U.S. Budget: Federal Trust Funds and the Politics of Commitment.* Cambridge: Cambridge University Press.

Pear, Robert (1993). "Health Aides Plan to Place Medicare Under New System.: *New York Times*, May 11, pp. A1, A16.

Pear, Robert (1999). "Government Says HMOs Mislead Medicare Recipients." *New York Times*, April 13, p. A18.

Perot, R. (1996). Address to the National Press Club. CNN Transcript #96102401V90, October 24.

Peterson, M. A. (1995). "Interest Groups as Allies and Antagonists: Their Role in the Politics of Health Care Reform." Paper prepared for delivery at the Annual Meeting of the Association for Health Services Research and Foundation for Health Services Research, Chicago, p. 13.

Peterson, M. A. (1998). "The Politics of Health Care Policy: Overreaching in an Age of Polarization." In Margaret Weir (Ed.), *The Social Divide: Political Parties and the Future of Activist Government* (pp. 181–229). Washington, DC: Brookings Institution Press.

Pham, Alex (1999). "Sweeping Medicare Overhaul is Planned." *Boston Globe*, February 28, pp. A1, A14.

President's Commission for a National Agenda for the Eighties (1990). *Report of the President's Commission for a National Agenda for the Eighties.* Washington, DC: U.S. Government Printing Office.

President's Midsession Review, July 24, 1992.

Prospective Payment Assessment Commission (PROPAC) (1992). *Medicare and the American Health Care System: Report and Recommendations to Congress.* Washington, DC: Author.

Quadagno, J. (1989). "Generational Equity and the Politics of the Welfare State." *Politics and Society* 17(3):353–76.

Reinhardt, U. E. (1997). "Medicare." New Members Issues Seminar, Congressional Research Service, January 21.

Rich, R. and W. D. White (1996). "National Health Reform: Where Do We Go from Here?" In R. Rich and W. D. White (Eds.), *Health Policy, Federalism and the American States.* Washington, DC: Urban Institute Press.

Rovner, J. (1987). "Democratic Leaders Slow Pace of Medicare Bill." *Congressional Quarterly Weekly Report* 45(27):1437–38.

Rushefsky, M. and K. Patel (1998). *Politics, Power and Policy Making: The Case of Health Care Reform in the 1990s.* Armonk, NY: M.E. Sharpe.

Schlesinger, M. and P. B. Drumheller (1988). "Beneficiary Cost Sharing in the Medicare Program." In D. Blumenthal, M. Schlesinger, and P. Drumheller

(Eds.), *Renewing the Promise: Medicare, Its History and Reform*. New York: Oxford University Press.

Skidmore, M. J. (1970). *Medicare and the American Rhetoric of Reconciliation*. Tuscaloosa: University of Alabama Press.

Skocpol, T. (1997). *Boomerang Health Care Reform and the Turn Against Government*. New York: W. W. Norton.

Smith, D. G. (1992). *Paying for Medicare: The Politics of Reform*. Hawthorne, NY: Aldine de Gruyter.

Smithey, Richard W. and T. R. Marmor (1987). "Understanding Medicare: Different Perspectives, An Essay Review." *Journal of the History of Medicine and Allied Sciences* 42(1):83–88.

Somers, H. M. and A. R. Somers (1967). *Medicare and the Hospitals: Issues and Prospects*. Washington, DC: Brookings Institution.

Starr, Paul (1982). *The Social Transformation of American Medicine*. New York: Basic Books.

Steinmo, S. and J. Watts (1995). "It's the Institutions, Stupid! Why Comprehensive National Health Insurance Always Fails in America." *Journal of Health Politics, Policy and Law* 20(Summer, 2):329–72.

Stevens, Rosemary (1989). *In Sickness and in Wealth: American Hospitals in the Twentieth Century*. New York: Basic Books.

Thorpe, K. (1992). "The Impact of Health Care Costs on the American Economy." Working paper, School of Public Health, University of North Carolina at Chapel Hill, August 31.

Tuohy, C. (1999). *Accidental Logics*. New York: Oxford University Press.

U.S. Bureau of the Census (1990). *Statistical Abstract of the United States, 1990*. Washington, DC: U.S. Government Printing Office.

U.S. Senate, Committee on Finance (1970). *Medicare and Medicaid: Problems, Issues, and Alternatives*. Report of the staff to the committee, February 9.

Washington Post (1996). "Rising Hospital Admissions Threaten Medical Fund." May 1, p. A17.

Weissert, C. S. and W. G. Weissert (1996). *Governing Health: The Politics of Health Policy*. Baltimore, MD: Johns Hopkins University Press.

White, J. (1995). "The Horses and the Jumps: Comments on the Health Care Reform Steeplechase." *Journal of Health Politics, Policy and Law* 20(Summer):373–84.

White, J. (1998). "'Saving' Medicare—From What?" Paper prepared for delivery at the Annual Meeting of the American Political Science Association, September 3–6. [Will be published in a report in *The Century Foundation, Understanding Long-Term Medicare Cost Estimates*.]

Yankelovich, D. (1995). "The Debate That Wasn't: The Public and the Clinton Health Plan." In Henry J. Aaron (Ed.), *The Problem That Won't Go Away: Reforming U.S. Health Care Financing* (Chapter 4). Washington, DC: Brookings Institution.

Index

AALL, 4–5
Aaron, H. J., 190–191
AARP, 134, 141
Access to medical care, 159
Accommodation, politics of, 55–56, 96–99, 172
Accretionist strategy, 57–58
Aetna Life Insurance Company, 48
AFDC, 82
AFL-CIO, 18–21, 39, 68, 73, 77
Aged, focus on, 10–15
Alford, Dale, 35–36
Alger, Bruce, 43
Allison, Graham T., 65, 174, 189
AMA (see American Medical Association)
American Association for Labor Legislation (AALL), 4–5
American Association of Retired Persons (AARP), 134, 141
American Hospital Association, 51, 54, 92
American Medical Association (AMA)
  disillusionment with, 116
  Douglas amendment and, 54
  Eldercare bill of, 46–53
  health insurance and, 5–6, 8–9, 15
  hospital insurance and, 15, 17–18
  House of Delegates, 5
  Kennedy administration versus, 38–44
  Kerr-Mills bill and, 29
  Medicare and, 17–21, 58, 60–61, 68, 74, 77–78
  premium support and, 177
  reform of Medicare and, 141
  voucher system and, 148, 177

American medical care system (Clinton proposal), 133–134
Americans for Generational Equity (1990), 131
AMPAC, 20
Anderson, Clinton, 31–32, 46, 54–55, 69
Annis, Edward, 79
Antigovernment sentiment, 159–160
Antiregulatory sentiment, 159–160
Antitrust sentiment, 161–162
Appel, James, 88

Baker, Russell, 37
Balanced Budget Act (1997), 141, 143–144, 147, 176
Ball, Robert, 16, 24, 77–79
Bankruptcy projections, 93–94, 123, 128, 132, 135–137, 142, 178
Baxter-Travenol and American Hospital Supply, 116
Bipartisan Commission on the Future of Medicare, 147, 162, 176–177
Blue Cross and Blue Shield, 6, 51, 73, 89, 107
Bowen, Otis, 110
Breaux, John, 147
Breaux-Thomas plan, 147–148, 187
Brown, Judith, 134
Brown, Larry, 113, 172, 186–187, 189
Budget deficit, federal, 123–124, 131
Bureaucratic politics, 174
Bush administration, 166, 175–176
Bush campaign (1992), 125
Bush, George, 126

Byrnes bill, 48–50
Byrnes, John W., 42, 48–50, 69

Canada's national health insurance
  system, 95, 132–133
Carter administration, 102
Case studies
  conceptual models and, 64
  knowledge and, cumulative, 63
  Medicare, 64, 71–80
  organizational process model and,
    67–69
  politics model and, 69–71
  rational actor model and, 64–67
Catastrophic health insurance, 24,
  112, 127
CBO, 125, 128
CHIP, 99
Civil Rights Act (1964), 88
Class conflicts, 19, 73–75
Clinton administration, 126–135, 172
Clinton, Bill, 127, 131, 133, 139,
  145–146, 148–149, 164
Clinton campaign (1992), 124–125
Clinton's national insurance reform,
  167
Cohen, Wilbur J., 9–11, 17, 23–24,
  29–30, 31, 38, 42, 49, 67, 69,
  77–78
Coinsurance, 50
Columbia HCA, 167–168
Commission on the Health Needs of
  the Nation (1952), 6–7, 13
Committee on Economic Security,
  5–6
Committee on National Health
  Insurance, 92
Committee on Political Education
  (COPE), 20
Competitive models of cost control,
  177
Comprehensive Health Insurance
  Plan (CHIP), 99
Conceptual models, 64
Concord Coalition (1992), 131
Congress
  81st, 8

87th, 30, 33–35
88th, 33–35, 71
89th, 53
Congressional Budget Office (CBO),
  125, 128
Congressional Quarterly (nonparti-
  san publication), 33, 44
Consumer sovereignty, 160–161
Contract with America, 139
COPE, 20
Corry, Martin, 127
Cost containment strategies, 102,
  108, 119, 127–128, 148, 175–177
Costs (see Expenditures)
Cruikshank, Nelson, 24, 78–79
Curtis, Thomas, 46
Customary costs, 97, 128

Daniels, Norman, 155
Darman plan, 125
Darman, Richard, 123
David, Sheri, 184
Deductibles, 50
Demystification of medical profes-
  sion, 163
Department of Health, Education,
  and Welfare (HEW), 42, 46, 53,
  75, 83–84, 91–92
Diagnosis-related group (DRG)
  reform, 108–110, 113, 116, 175,
  187
Dingell (Senator), 7
Disability insurance, 24, 156
Dixon-Yates, 78, 80
Doctor visits, 3–4
Douglas, Paul, 54–55
DRG reform, 108–110, 113, 116, 175,
  187
Durenberger (Senator), 124

Edelman, Murray, 83
Eisenhower administration, 23–30
Eldercare bill, 46–53
Election years
  1964, 41, 45
  1992, 124–126
  1996, 172

Ellwood, Paul, 161
Evaluation of healthcare facilities, 88
Ewing, Oscar, 9–10, 15–16, 59
Expenditures
  customary costs, 97, 128
  health care, general, 4, 84, 89–91, 105–106, 163
  Medicare, 88–89, 102–104, 108, 111, 114, 128–131
  physician fees, 50, 54–55, 84, 89, 98, 108, 113, 116, 128
  RAPP specialists, 50, 54–55
  reasonable costs, 89, 97–98, 128
  Social Security, 16

Fair Deal, 6–11, 64, 67
Falk, I. S., 9–10, 24, 67
Feder, Judy, 187
Federal Security Agency, 11, 66
Federation of American Health Systems, 148, 177
Fee-for-service (FFS), 161
Forand, Aime, 24
Forand bill (1960), 24–27, 31–32, 36, 60, 81–82
Forand hearings, 24
Fraud, Medicare, 145–146
Frazier (Representative), 34, 36, 42
Friedman, Lawrence, 81–83
Fulton, Richard, 42

Gardner, John, 91
Generational equity, 131–132, 140, 155–156
Gingrich, Newt, 139
Golden Ring Clubs, 21
Gradualism (*see* Incrementalism, politics of)
Gramm-Rudman legislation (1985), 115
Great Depression, 5
Great Society, 46, 133, 145, 152
Griffiths, Martha, 34

Hacker, Jacob, 187
Harrison, Burr, 36–37, 42

Health Care Financing Administration (HCFA), 102, 104, 118, 148, 156, 175
Health insurance (*see also* Medicare)
  American Medical Association and, 5–6, 8–9, 15
  in Canada, 95, 132–133
  catastrophic, 24, 112, 127
  Clinton's national reform, 167
  coinsurance and, 50
  deductibles, 50
  in Great Britain, 12, 152
  growth of private, 111
  historical perspective of, 4
  incrementalism and, 16–17
  lobbyists and, 17–21
  Medigap plans and, 113, 125
  national strategies, 100–101
  purpose of general, 12
  universal government and, 4–6, 8–9
Health maintenance organizations (HMOs), 99, 102–103, 119, 161
Health Planning and Resources Development Act (1974), 101
Health systems agencies (HSAs), 101
Heinz, John, 125
Henderson, Lawrence, 3
Heritage Foundation proposal (1993), 166
Herlong, A. Sydney, 34, 36, 46
Herzlinger, Regina, 163
HEW, 42, 46, 53, 75, 83–84, 91–92
"High School Debate Kit" radio tapes and scripts, 39
HMOs, 99, 102–103, 119, 161
Hospital Corporations of America, 116
Hospital expenditures, 98
Hospital insurance, 12–13, 15, 17–18, 46, 55–56
Housing policy, 81–82
Howard, Ernest, 38–39, 46
H.R. 1, 46–53, 70
H.R. 3737, 46–53
H.R. 4222, 39
H.R. 4351, 48–50

H.R. 6675, 50–55
HSAs, 101
Humanas, 115–116
Hutton, William, 79

Idealogical context of Medicare's poli-
    tics
  background information on,
    151–152
  precompetitive movement and,
    152, 157–168
  roots of, philosophical, 152–157
Ikard, Frank, 34, 36, 42
Incrementalism, politics of, 10–11,
    16–17, 66, 96
Insider politics, 175–176
Insolvency projections, 93–94, 123,
    128, 132, 135–137, 142, 178
Insurance (see specific types)

Jacobs, Lawrence, 184–186, 189
Javits (Senator), 38
Jennings, Pat, 42
Johnson administration, 42–44,
    46–61, 91–92
Johnson, Lyndon B., 42, 56, 58, 91
Jost, Tim, 186

Kaiser-Permanente, 167–168
Keating, Kenneth, 39
Kennedy administration, 29–44
Kennedy, John F., 29–30, 35–38, 42,
    57
Kerr, Robert, 28–29, 32
Kerr-Mills bill (1960), 27–30, 32,
    48–49, 60, 76, 81–82, 99, 152
Key, V. O., 75
King, Cecil, 31–32, 46
King-Anderson bill (1961), 32, 35–40,
    42–44, 46, 49, 59, 61
Knowledge, cumulative, 63

Life expectancy, 3
Lobbyists, 17–21, 47, 68, 77–78 (see
    also specific names)
Long, Russell, 53–54, 69

Long-Ribicoff catastrophic plan, 99,
    161
Lowi, Theodore, 19, 72–73, 75, 78, 80

McCormack (Representative), 36–37
Machrowicz, Thaddeus, 34
McNamara, Pat, 28–29
Macro politics, 176–179
Major risk insurance (MRI), 161
Majoritarianism, 174
Managed care plans, 131, 144–145,
    177, 187
Market for medical care, 162–168
Marmor, T. R., 191
Mashaw, J., 191
MCCA (1988), 110, 112–113
Medicaid Anti-Fraud and Abuse
    Amendments (1977), 104
Medical progress, 3
Medical Savings Accounts, 144
Medicare (see also Politics of
    Medicare; Reform of Medicare)
  American Medical Association and,
    17–21, 58, 60–61, 68, 74, 77–78
  background information on, 4–6
  case studies, 64, 71–80
  Catastrophic Coverage Act (1988)
    and, 110, 112–113
  complexity of, 107
  confusion about, 104, 107
  cost containment, 102, 108, 119,
    127–128, 148, 175–176
  crises, 137, 158, 172
  current status, 151
  defeat of, initial, 38–44
  development, 154
  Douglas amendment and, 54–55
  enactment of, 4–5, 56, 69–71
  enrollment, initial, 87–88
  entitlement, 153–154
  evaluation of healthcare facilities
    and, 88
  evolution of, 96–99, 173–175
  expenditures, 88–89, 102–104, 108,
    111, 114, 128–131
  flip-flop, 147–149, 176

fraud, 145–146
generational equity and, 131–132, 140, 155–156
growth of, 100, 111, 156–157
Health Care Financing Administration and, 102, 104, 118, 148, 156, 175
H.R. 1 and, 46–53, 70
H.R. 6675 and, 50–55
implementation of, initial, 87–92, 96–99
insolvency projections and, 93–94, 123, 128, 132, 135–137, 142, 178
medical progress and, 4
origins of, 64–67, 95–96, 152
procompetitive movement and, 152, 158–162
progress of (1970s), 99–107
Reagan administration and, 107–116, 118
responses of (1952–64), 67–69
rider, 37–38
risk selection, 143–144
S. 1 and, 46–53
scholarship on, 183–191
terminology, 193–207
trust fund, 132, 135–136, 138
Ways and Means Committee and, 32–35, 41–42, 47
Medicare + Choice option, 143
Medicare Act of 1965, 4–5, 56, 59
Medicare Catastrophic Coverage Act (MCCA) (1988), 110, 112–113
Medicare Preservation Act (1995), 139
"The Medicare Reform Debate" (Aaron & Reischauer), 190
Medigap plans, 113, 125
Meranto, Philip, 75
Microeconomic approach to analyzing social policy, 159
Mills, Wilbur, 28–29, 32, 34–37, 40, 42–44, 48–53, 58, 60, 69–70, 137
Moon, Marilyn, 188–189
Morone, Jim, 187, 189
MRI, 161

Murray (Senator), 7
Murray-Wagner-Dingell bill (1949), 7–8, 15

National Academy of Social Insurance Task Force on Medicare, 191
National Bipartisan Commission on the Future of Medicare, 147, 162, 176–177
National Commission on Social Security Reform (1982), 110
National Committee to Preserve Social Security and Medicare, 112
National Council of Senior Citizens, 18, 21
National Health Service of Great Britain, 12, 152
New Deal, 5, 57, 133, 145
New Frontier, 31
New Republic (liberal weekly), 33, 53
Nixon administration, 161

OASI, 9, 15, 27
Oberlander, Jon, 137, 183, 186, 190
Old Age and Survivors Insurance system (OASI), 9, 15, 27
Oliver, Tom, 189
"Operation Hometown" campaign, 39
Organizational process model, 67–69

Paradox of medical progress, 3
Patel, K., 187
Permissive consensus, 75
Perot, Ross, 95
Peterson, Mark, 186
Peterson, Peter, 124
Physican fees, 50, 54–55, 84, 89, 98, 108, 113, 116, 128
Physician visits, 3–4
Physicians' service insurance, 52–53, 60
Political Action Committee of AMA (AMPAC), 20
Political conflict patterns, 72

Politics of Medicare (*see also* Ideolog-
     ical context of Medicare politics;
     specific laws)
  accommodation, 55–56, 96–99,
     172
  aged and, focus on, 10–15
  Bush administration and, 175–176
  Carter administration and, 102
  case studies, 64, 71–80
  class conflicts, 19, 73–75
  Clinton administration and,
     126–135, 139
  defeats of Medicare bill, initial,
     38–44
  Douglas amendment and, 54–55
  Eisenhower administration and,
     23–30
  election of 1964 and, 41, 45
  election of 1992 and, 124–126
  election of 1996 and, 172
  in evolution from 1966–70, 96–99
  expenditures, early, 96–99
  Fair Deal and, 6–11, 64, 67
  H.R. 1 and, 46–53, 70
  H.R. 6675 and, 50–55
  ideological context of, 151–168
  implementation, initial, 96–99
  incrementalism, 10–11, 16–17, 66,
     96
  insider, 175–176
  Johnson administration and,
     42–44, 46–61
  Kennedy administration and,
     29–42
  lessons of, 56–61
  literature on administrative
     (1966–99), 185–191
  lobbyists and, 17–21, 47, 68, 77–78
  macro, 176–179
  majoritarianism, 174
  in 1970s, 99–107
  in 1980s, 107–115
  in 1990s, 123, 172
  overview from 1966–99, 93–94,
     115–119
  patterns and puzzles in, under-
     standing, 171–180

Reagan administration and,
     107–116, 118, 175–176
  reform and, 123–124
  S. 1 and, 46–53
  Senate and House Conference
     Committee and, 55–56
  social policy and, character of,
     80–85
  Social Security contributors and,
     focus on, 15–17
  southern Democrats and, 35–38, 40
  Truman administration and, 6–11,
     17–18, 60, 64, 66–67
Politics model, 69–71
Poor Laws, 16, 131
PPGP, 161
Premium support, 177
Prepaid group practices (PPGP), 161
Pressure groups, 17–21, 47, 68, 77–78
     (*see also specific names*)
Price controls, 102, 108, 119,
     127–128, 148, 175, 175–177
Procompetitive movement
  market for medical care and,
     162–168
  Medicare and, 152, 158–162
  rise of, 157–158
Professional standards review organ-
     izations (PSROs), 99
Public Law 86–778, 27–30
Public Law 89–97, 4–5, 56, 59
Public Law 93641, 101
Public Law 95142, 104
Public opinion, mass, 75
Public policy (*see* Social policy)

Quealy, William, 48

Rangel, Charles, 139
Ranney, Austin, 80–81
RAPP specialists, 50, 54–55
Rational actor model, 64–67
Rayburn (Representative), 36–37
RBRVS, 108, 113, 116
Reagan administration, 107–116,
     118, 175–176
Reasonable costs, 89, 97–98, 128

Reform of Medicare
  American Association of Retired
    Persons and, 141
  American Medical Association and,
    141
  Balanced Budget Act (1997) and,
    141, 143–144, 147
  budget deficit and, federal,
    123–124, 131
  Bush administration and, 166
  Clinton administration's strategy
    for, 133–135, 139, 167
  cost containment, 127–128,
    132–135
  diagnosis-related group, 108–110,
    113, 116, 175, 187
  election of 1992 and, 124–126
  generational equity, 155–156
  legacy of, 166–168
  Medicare + Choice option, 143
  negative consensus of, 126–135
  in 1970s, 99–107
  in 1990s, 123–149
  in 1997, 124, 137–147
  physician fees, 108, 113, 116,
    128
  politics of, 123–124
  in Reagan era, 107–115
  Republican (1995), 139–140
  Trustees Report (1995) and,
    135–137
Regulation of industry, government,
  116
Reischauer, R.D., 190–191
*Report of the President's Commission
  for a National Agenda for the
  Eighties* (1980), 160
Resource Based Relative Value Scale
  (RBRVS), 108, 113, 116
Ribicoff, Abraham, 39–40
Rider, Medicare, 37–38
Risk selection, 143–144
Roosevelt, Franklin Delano, 5–6,
  57
Rostenkowski, Dan, 112
Rudman, (Senator), 124
Rushevsky, K., 187

S 1, 46–53
Scholarship on Medicare, 183–191
Schultze, Charles, 159
Senate Committee on Aging, 29
Senate Finance Committee, 28,
  53–55
Senate and House Conference Com-
  mittee (1965), 55–56
Senior Citizens' Councils, 18, 21
Skocpol, Theda, 189
Smith, David, 187
Social policy (*see also* Medicare)
  changes in, timing of, 145
  character of, 80–85
  housing, 81–82
  Medicare case and, 71–80
  microeconomic approach to analyz-
    ing, 159
  political conflict in, patterns of, 72
  public opinion and, mass, 75
Social Security Act (1935), 5–6, 9,
  51–52, 81
Social Security Administration
  (SSA), 16, 83–85, 87–88, 91, 97
Social Security Amendments (1972),
  99, 102
Social Security approach to health
  care, 25–28, 84–85
Social Security contributors, focus
  on, 15–17
Socialism, 39, 92, 165
Somers, Anne, 3
Somers, Herman, 3
Southern Democrats, 35–38, 40
Special interest groups, 17–21, 47,
  68, 77–78 (*see also specific
  names*)
SSA, 16, 83–85, 87–88, 91, 97
Stark (Representative), 141
Starr, Paul, 189
Stowe, David, 10
Supplementary Medical Insurance
  Program, 87

Thomas, Bill, 147–148
Thompson, Clark, 34, 42
Thornburgh, Richard, 126

Truman administration, 6–11, 17–18, 60, 64, 66–67

Truman, Harry, 6–11

Trust funds, 16, 132, 135–136, 138

Trustees Report (1995), 135–137

Tsongas (Senator), 124

Unitary Actor Model, 189

Voucher system, 148, 177

Wagner, Robert, 7

Watts, John, 36

Ways and Means Committee
  H.R. 1 and, 47–53
  H.R. 6675 and, 51–55
  King-Anderson bill and, 39, 43

Medicare and, 32–35, 41–42, 47
  in 1961, 33–35
  in 1965, 45

Weissert, Carol, 187

Weissert, William, 187

Welfare approach to health care, 25–28, 96

Whitaker and Baxter (public relations firm), 8

Wicker, Tom, 52

Wilcox, Alanson, 54

Wildavsky, Aaron, 19, 78, 80

Witte, Edwin, 5–6

Wofford, Harris, 125–126

Wolkstein, Irwin, 50, 59, 78–79

Yale Law Journal study, 41